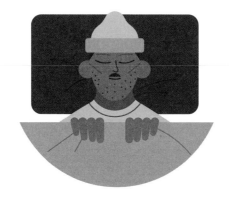

the

SCIENCE

of

SLEEP

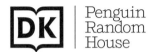

Project Editor Aimée Longos
Project Designer Alison Gardner
Editor Andrea Page
Senior Editor Rona Skene
US Editor Kayla Dugger
Senior Art Editor Barbara Zuniga
Jacket Designer Amy Cox
Jackets Coordinator Lucy Philpott
Pre-production Producer Heather Blagden
Senior Production Controller Luca Bazzoli
Managing Editor Dawn Henderson
Managing Art Editor Marianne Markham
Art Director Maxine Pedliham
Publishing Director Katie Cowan

Illustrator Owen Davey

First American Edition, 2021
Published in the United States by DK Publishing
1450 Broadway, Suite 801, New York, NY 10018

DISCLAIMER see page 224

A catalog record for this book
is available from the Library of Congress.
ISBN 978-0-7440-3368-7

Printed and bound in China

For the curious
www.dk.com

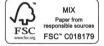

the
SCIENCE
of
SLEEP

Stop chasing a good night's sleep and let it find you

HEATHER DARWALL-SMITH

Contents

MIND AND BODY 64

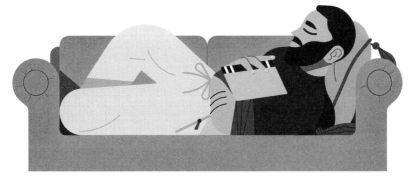

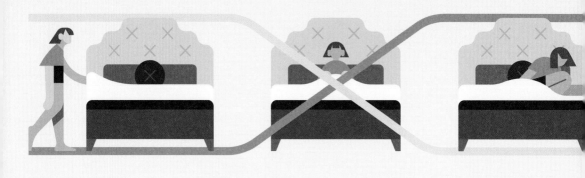

Foreword

I am fascinated by sleep; it is the ultimate act of "letting go." It's also something we tend to take for granted—until problems occur. Suddenly, sleep becomes a fruitless endeavor, and the more we chase it, the more elusive it becomes. Our fixation on perfect sleep interferes with our very ability to achieve it.

As a sleep psychotherapist, my approach is to ask patients to implement various processes to improve their sleep and to explain exactly how and why these strategies work. I feel strongly that everyone should have access to this knowledge, and that's why I wanted to write this book.

I know that, as human beings, we are biologically programmed to be able to sleep—and by working through all the factors that might get in the way of this instinct, each of us can figure out what we need to do in order to be able to prioritize sleep and regain the knack of letting it come naturally.

This book is for anyone who wants to learn about sleep, avoiding the misleading and sometimes harmful clamor that often accompanies the topic. It will guide you through the basics of what sleep is and how it works, then address the most important issues we have around sleep—based on questions

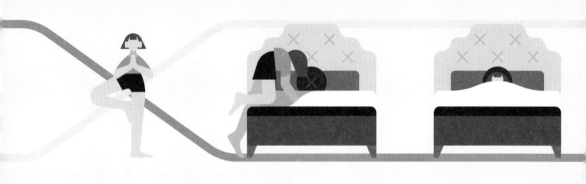

I am asked on a daily basis in my practice. These are divided into easy-to-digest sections covering all the factors that can influence the quality and quantity of your sleep, including physical and mental health, age, lifestyle, and your sleep environment.

Sleep science is a dynamic, diverse field encompassing every aspect of our biology. New discoveries are constantly being made as we work on unraveling the mysteries of sleep. I continue to study to be able to include the latest findings in my day-to-day work with clients.

Perhaps the most important message I can share with you is that no one sleeps perfectly—and that's okay. My mission in this book is to help you understand and work with your own sleep profile, which is as unique as your fingerprint. Sleep is a vital piece in the jigsaw puzzle of health and well-being—and by balancing factors such as getting enough sunlight, staying active, reducing stress, and eating well, you really can help yourself to a good night's sleep.

Sleep well—and sweet dreams.

Heather Darwall-Smith

Heather Darwall-Smith

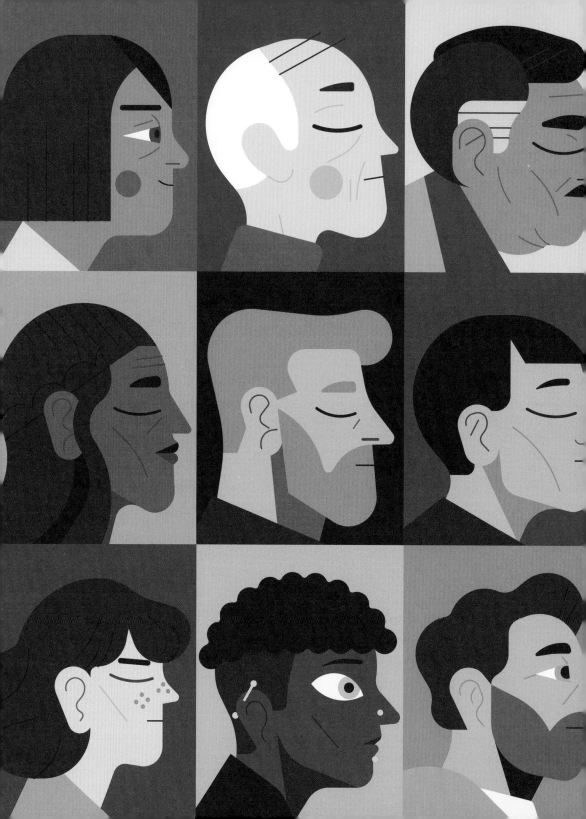

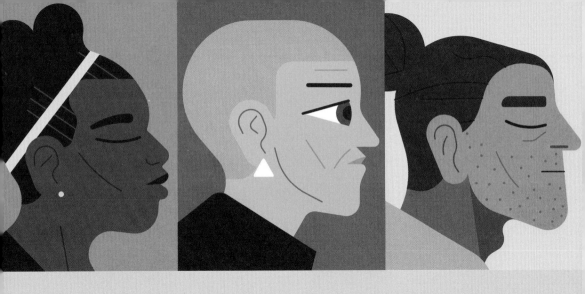

SLEEP BASICS

There are new discoveries every day about how and why we sleep—but everything scientists learn confirms that this seemingly simple function lies at the heart of our health and well-being.

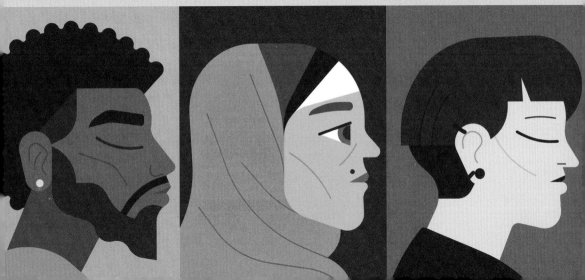

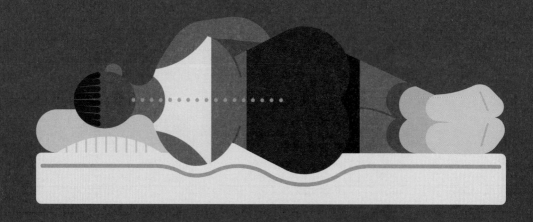

The simple truth about sleep

There's still much we don't know about sleep, and understanding exactly what it is and why we need it can feel difficult. Cutting through the jargon and coming to grips with some simple scientific principles will help you understand more about this vital process.

What is sleep, and why do we need it?

Sleep is amazing in ways that science has only recently begun to discover. That we spend so much of our lives doing it potentially highlights the biological importance of sleep.

When we sleep, we enter a specific state that lies somewhere between consciousness and unconsciousness—the body is at rest, but the brain remains highly active and hard at work. Sleep is vital for our survival, and a whole range of biological functions can only be undertaken while we are in this state. Scientists are discovering more all the time, but the main functions of sleep seem to be: diverting energy into clearing harmful toxins from the brain and body, consolidating learning and memory, boosting the immune system, balancing our emotional states, and repairing and restoring cells in the body. These rejuvenation processes are essential for us to function optimally, and when we sleep well, our mental, cognitive, and physical health are all dramatically improved.

Although many of the mysteries of sleep remain unknown, what is becoming increasingly clear is that sleep is essential to our well-being and that in order to live well, we must take it as seriously as we take eating and exercise. The more science uncovers, the more we understand that good sleep holds the keys to health and happiness.

Apart from its biological function, consistent good sleep, quite simply, feels great. By understanding sleep's importance and how to improve it, it's possible to let go of worrying about it, get into bed, and just drift off.

The brain and body in sleep
While we sleep, the brain and body undergo a series of repair and consolidation processes that affect every aspect of our functioning.

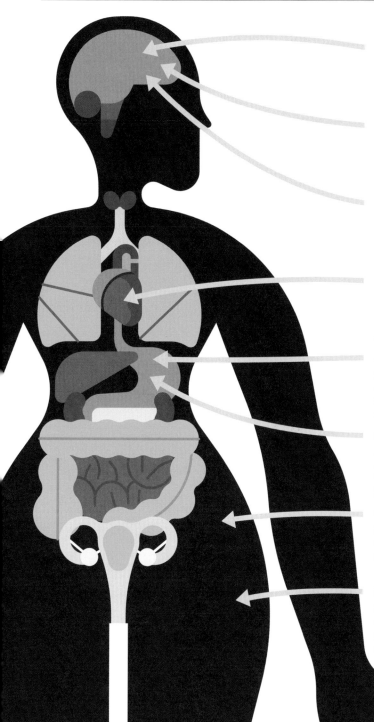

Mood

Sleep regulates mood; good sleep gives the brain's emotional center the chance to rest, leaving us feeling positive and upbeat on waking.

Detoxification and rest

The brain signals muscles to relax as we sleep. It also runs waste-clearance processes to remove harmful proteins that have built up during the day.

Memory and learning

As we sleep, the brain processes our experiences from the day, deciding what needs storing and what doesn't.

Heart and blood pressure

Blood pressure drops overnight in order to decrease the strain on the heart and blood vessels, helping reduce the risk of cardiovascular disease.

Appetite

Sleep regulates the hormones that control hunger and fullness signals, helping us eat appropriate amounts and manage our weight.

Immunity

As we sleep, we produce defenses such as T-cells to fight infections and viruses. We also make proteins that fight inflammation.

Growth

Human growth hormone is released, which repairs cell damage and strengthens bones and muscles.

Cell repair and skin

Getting enough sleep means that antioxidants are released, which help repair cells and skin damage and reduce inflammation.

The history of the science of sleep

Only since the turn of the 20th century and the development of ways to measure brain activity during sleep has sleep begun to be more widely understood. The 1950s heralded what is now a standalone discipline—the science of sleep.

Timeline of key discoveries in sleep science

1845
First connection made between human body temperature and sleep patterns

1888
Data documenting narcolepsy (see page 52) first published

1899
Sigmund Freud's *Interpretation of Dreams* is published, outlining a theory of dream analysis

1922
Identification of hypothalamus as the area of the brain responsible for regulating sleep/wake cycles

1972
The suprachiasmatic nucleus (SCN, see pages 22–23), in the hypothalamus, identified as seat of the circadian clock

1971
Period gene (PER) identified as playing a role in the timings of behaviors such as waking in circadian rhythm

1970
First sleep laboratory focusing on sleep disorders opens at Stanford University

1966
"The bunker experiment" indicates a natural 24-hour rhythm exists even when not exposed to daylight

1973
Cognitive Behavioral Therapy (CBT) first used as a treatment for insomnia

1979
Treatment known as continuous positive airway pressure (CPAP) for sleep apnea is first used

1982
Two-process model of sleep homeostasis (Process S) and the circadian clock (Process C) proposed

2003
Theory proposed linking homeostatic sleep regulation to learning

The mystery of sleep has been of interest to physicians, scientists, and philosophers as far back as around 350 BCE, when the Ancient Greeks considered sleep to be a type of physiological state somehow related to digestion. Since the discovery of sleeping brainwaves in the 1930s, the science of sleep has progressed at great speed, with huge advances and achievements in our understanding of the mechanics of sleep.

1937
Using recording of brain waves by electro-encephalogram (EEG), five sleep stages identified

1950s
Polysomnography—an in-depth sleep study practice—established, using EEGs and other markers

1951–1953
Discovery of rapid eye movement (REM) sleep, a light sleep phase in which vivid dreams occur

1956
Obstructive sleep apnea (OSA, see page 75) first described and classified

1962
The pons region of the brain is identified as controlling REM sleep

1960
The term "zeitgeber" coined to describe external cues the body uses to synchronize its circadian cycle

1959
The term "circadian" (Latin for "about a day") first used to describe the body's sleep/wake rhythms

1958
Discovery of the hormone melatonin as being responsible for regulating the sleep/wake cycle

2005
US National Institute of Health suggests CBT as the first-line treatment for insomnia

2009
DEC2 gene discovered showing that short sleep duration is genetic for those with this mutation

2017
Nobel Prize awarded to a team that uncovered molecular mechanisms controlling the circadian rhythm

2017
Discovery of "insomnia gene" Crypto-chrome 1 (CRY1), which can disrupt the body's natural rhythms

The quantity of sleep we need

It's a myth that everyone requires exactly eight hours of sleep a night—your sleep needs are personal and can depend on a variety of factors, in particular your age.

Aside from age, other biological factors may influence your sleep needs, such as your state of health and whether you are taking any medications. However, quantity is only half the story—external factors such as work, family life, and your lifestyle can also affect how well you sleep, so you may not feel fully rested and refreshed even when you do get your full "quota" of hours.

What's the recommendation for my age?
Studies have shown that many of us get far less sleep than we need to function at our best, and in recent years, scientists have updated their recommendations to reflect these findings. In the US, for instance, the National Sleep Foundation issued new guidelines in 2015 for the amount of sleep different age groups require—with the suggested number of hours increasing in almost half of the age categories. The revised guidelines also saw the addition of two new age categories: younger adults and older

adults. While much is known about the changes in sleep as we age, little is understood about the sleep needs of young adults. Early adulthood is an important developmental period, one marked by a transition into the workplace where alertness and productivity can become significantly impacted by sleep deprivation. Research to learn more about sleep needs for this age group is ongoing.

The right amount of sleep for you
As well as using your age as a guide to how much sleep you need, a sleep journal (see pages 36–37) can help you determine if you are getting enough slumber. As a rule of thumb, if you are often drowsy during the day or find yourself reaching for a quick caffeine fix in the afternoon, you probably need more sleep. Once you understand your own needs, you can work on creating a routine to get the right amount of sleep for your individual circumstances.

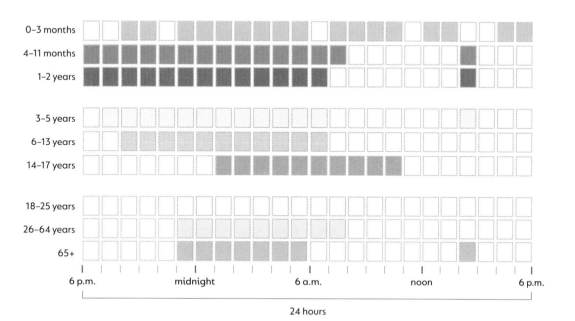

| | 6 p.m. | midnight | 6 a.m. | noon | 6 p.m. |

24 hours

Sleep needs by age group

The amount of nightly sleep we need changes as we age. Newborns require the most sleep, at around 17 hours, and older adults the least, but everyone needs at least 6 hours.

0–3 months

Newborns' sleep patterns are irregular, but they sleep for the majority of the day to allow for vital growth and development.

3–5 years

Sleep needs drop by around an hour and napping comes to an end, but nighttime waking is still common.

18–25 years

After puberty finishes, the body clock shifts back again. Young adults need slightly less sleep than teenagers.

4–11 months

Infants' sleep patterns become more regular, but overall sleep needs remain high to allow for continued growth.

6–13 years

Sleep needs are still high, but school requirements and extracurricular activities mean bedtime becomes slightly later.

26–64 years

Sleep needs remain steady in working-age people, aiding alertness, daily routines, and productivity.

1–2 years

Toddlers sleep slightly less than infants; mastery of new skills along with teething can mean they often fight sleep.

14–17 years

A shift in the body clock means that teenagers need to sleep later but often are unable to do so due to school timetables.

65+

Hormonal changes and less need for growth and cell replenishment mean we need less sleep in old age, but napping returns.

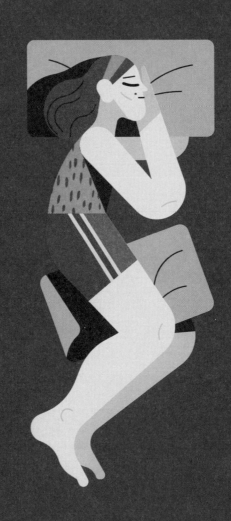

The mechanics of good sleep

Your amazing body knows what it needs to do in order to get the sleep necessary to keep it in great working order. Every day, it orchestrates a series of intricate processes that work together like cogs in a machine to help you sleep and wake at the right times.

The body's circadian rhythm

Your body knows instinctively when to sleep due to its internal clock—its "circadian rhythm." This clock regulates the timing of all our functions on an approximate 24-hour cycle.

Our circadian rhythm is what regulates the timings of sleep, as well as many other aspects of our biological functioning and behavior. Derived from the Latin *circa*, meaning "about," and *dies*, meaning "a day," this circadian rhythm is known as "Process C," and it is the master clock that keeps all our bodily systems ticking along and working in harmony with one another.

Governed by light

The master clock is controlled by an area of the brain called the suprachiasmatic nucleus (SCN), a cluster of 20,000 neurons found in the hypothalamus. The SCN is reset each day by daylight—our eyes track the changing light levels and signal the SCN to synchronize our internal clock to match the rhythm of the external environment and to trigger various bodily functions in response to these cues.

Process C is essential for humans to function; it controls vital actions such as the regulation of body temperature, digestion, and the production of various hormones. Any changes to the external cues we receive—for example, in the amount of light we get—can therefore confuse Process C and disrupt the natural rhythm of our bodies. Living in harmony with our circadian clock is a key component of good health, and sleeping well is one of the most important factors in keeping Process C on track.

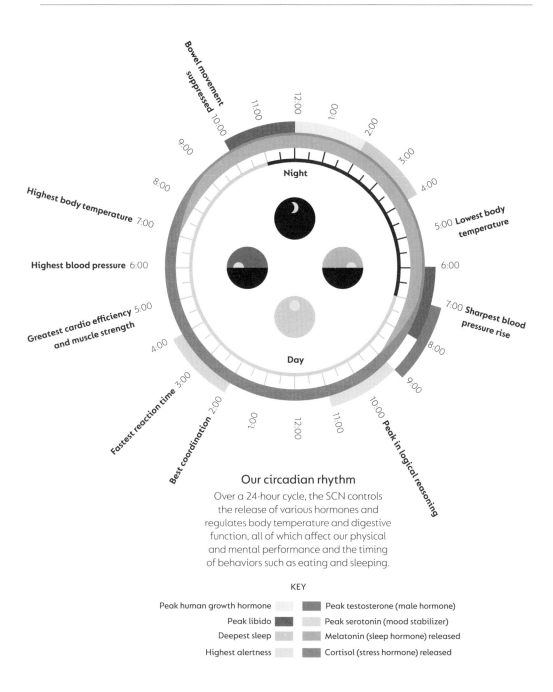

Our circadian rhythm

Over a 24-hour cycle, the SCN controls
the release of various hormones and
regulates body temperature and digestive
function, all of which affect our physical
and mental performance and the timing
of behaviors such as eating and sleeping.

KEY

Peak human growth hormone	Peak testosterone (male hormone)
Peak libido	Peak serotonin (mood stabilizer)
Deepest sleep	Melatonin (sleep hormone) released
Highest alertness	Cortisol (stress hormone) released

Bowel movement suppressed 10:00
11:00
12:00
1:00
2:00
3:00
4:00
5:00 Lowest body temperature
6:00
7:00 Sharpest blood pressure rise
8:00
9:00
10:00 Peak in logical reasoning
11:00
12:00
1:00
Best coordination 2:00
Fastest reaction time 3:00
4:00
Greatest cardio efficiency and muscle strength 5:00
Highest blood pressure 6:00
Highest body temperature 7:00
8:00
9:00

Night

Day

The sleep/wake cycle

Our rhythm of sleeping and waking is regulated by two biological processes that work together: our circadian rhythm (Process C) and our homeostatic sleep pressure (Process S). This is known as the two-process model of sleep.

Our sleep pressure—the urge to go to sleep—increases over the course of the day, and the longer we stay awake, the greater this will be. Although this process is still not fully understood, what is known is that the pressure to sleep comes from the build-up in the brain of adenosine, a chemical that encourages drowsiness. The rise and fall of sleep pressure over a 24-hour period is called the homeostatic process, or "Process S."

However, even when sleep pressure has built up, it may not always mean it's easy to fall asleep. This is because our circadian rhythm—Process C (see pages 22–23)—also plays a significant part in dictating the timing of when we fall asleep. When the circadian clock signals that it's time for sleep, sleep pressure peaks and our "sleep gate" opens—the doorway to the sleep zone.

When Process C and Process S are synchronized, your sleep/wake cycle runs smoothly; as you sleep, adenosine is gradually broken down, and Process C triggers the release of the sleep-inducing hormone melatonin. As morning approaches, Process C triggers the release of alertness hormones to wake you. However, if processes C and S are out of sync—for example, if your caffeine consumption blocks adenosine (see pages 154–155)—this can lead to problems such as difficulty falling or staying asleep or waking too early.

Regulating the sleep/wake cycle

The mechanism that moves us between sleep and wakefulness is known as the "flip-flop switch"—a system that controls the brain circuitry via two nerve cell groups. One group wakes us and the other sends us to sleep, but only one group can be active at any given time. The flipping of this switch is controlled by the neurotransmitter orexin. If the sleep switch is damaged, for example, by a brain injury, or if levels of orexin are too low, such as in those with narcolepsy (see page 52), the ability to move between sleep and wakefulness can become unstable, leading to a range of sleep disorders.

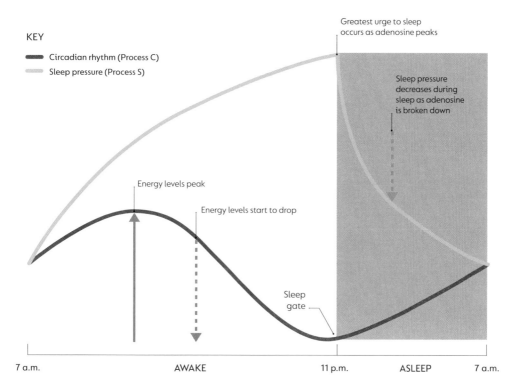

KEY

━━ Circadian rhythm (Process C)
━━ Sleep pressure (Process S)

Greatest urge to sleep
occurs as adenosine peaks

Sleep pressure
decreases during
sleep as adenosine
is broken down

Energy levels peak

Energy levels start to drop

Sleep
gate

7 a.m.   AWAKE   11 p.m.   ASLEEP   7 a.m.

Sleep pressure

The pressure to sleep increases over the course of
the day as adenosine levels rise, taking cues for
sleepiness from Process C, until you can resist no
more and you are pushed through the "sleep gate"
and fall asleep at night.

Hormones and sleep

Hormones are chemical messengers that travel in the bloodstream and trigger certain bodily functions. Several hormones are associated with our circadian rhythm and regulating the sleep/wake cycle.

The levels of certain hormones in the body fluctuate throughout the day in response to our circadian rhythm, telling us, for instance, when to feel sleepy and when to wake up. Although some hormones directly regulate sleep, the relationship between hormones and sleep is a two-way street: the production of hormones, and the impact this has on sleep patterns, can also be influenced by the quality and quantity of our sleep.

Melatonin
Pineal gland

The "sleepiness" hormone helps build our sleep pressure and decrease body temperature, both necessary for us to be able to fall asleep and stay asleep.

Cortisol
Adrenal gland

The "stress" hormone increases alertness, so it peaks in the early morning. It is also triggered as part of the body's "fight-or-flight" stress response to threatening situations.

Progesterone
Ovaries and adrenal gland

Progesterone affects body temperature, REM sleep, and levels of gamma-aminobutyric acid—which can induce relaxation and sleepiness.

Serotonin
Pineal gland and the gut

The "happy" hormone's main job is to regulate mood and maintain wakefulness, but serotonin is also turned into melatonin, which is vital for inducing sleep.

Human growth hormone
Pituitary gland

This hormone is released in pulses during deep sleep. It plays a vital role in muscle and tissue repair and metabolism.

Aldosterone
Outer adrenal glands

This hormone acts to regulate sodium and potassium in the blood. High levels secreted during sleep help prevent you from needing to urinate at night.

Oxytocin
Hypothalamus and pituitary gland

The "love" hormone is important for social and sexual behavior and slows the nervous system to promote sleep.

HORMONES OF THE SLEEP/WAKE CYCLE

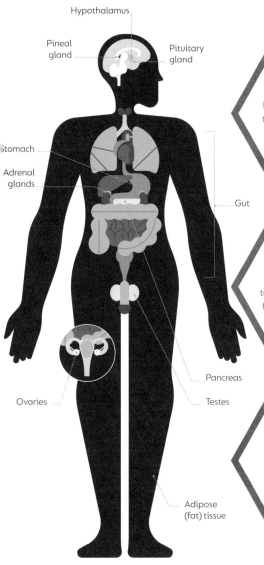

Hypothalamus

Pineal gland

Pituitary gland

Stomach

Adrenal glands

Gut

Ovaries

Pancreas

Testes

Adipose (fat) tissue

Prolactin
Pituitary gland

Hormone involved in the immune response, along with the production of breast milk. Most prolactin is secreted during deep sleep, so good sleep ensures successful release.

Adrenaline
Adrenal glands

Hormone produced as part of the body's stress response. Raised levels of adrenaline can block the ability to fall asleep, so avoiding too much stress before bedtime is key for sleep quality.

Testosterone
Testes

Made in the testes, ovaries, and adrenal glands, testosterone affects libido and fertility. Release peaks during sleep, so good shut-eye is key to sexual and reproductive health.

Ghrelin and leptin
Fat tissue and stomach

Leptin is produced in the fat tissues, and ghrelin in the stomach. These hormones control hunger and fullness, and good sleep keeps them well-balanced.

Insulin
Pancreas

This hormone regulates blood sugar levels. Some of this vital process takes place in deep sleep, so sleeping well helps keep blood sugar levels in a healthy range.

**OTHER HORMONES
AFFECTED BY SLEEP**

The stages of sleep

Sleep is not a static state—quite the opposite. Once asleep, the body begins its processes of rest and repair, passing through several distinct stages to do so. It does this in cycles, which repeat these stages around four or five times each night.

Sleep scientists identify four stages of sleep: three stages of non-REM sleep; Stage-1 (NREM 1) and Stage-2 (NREM 2) light sleep; and Stage-3 (NREM 3) deep sleep, which is also known as slow-wave sleep (SWS); then a fourth stage of rapid eye movement (REM) sleep. Each stage has unique features that allow the body and brain to carry out essential processes to prepare them for the next day. Stage-1 sleep occurs as you transition from wakefulness to sleep. During this stage, you can be easily awakened by external stimuli. Stage-2 sleep is also light, but this is when the brain fires sleep spindles—bursts of activity thought to be involved in memory consolidation, which also prevent you from waking. During Stage-3 sleep, you are much

less easily roused, but if you are, you are often disoriented. Stage 3 is also when most of the brain and body's repair processes take place. During the REM stage of sleep,

Rapid eye movement

REM sleep occurs in all sleep cycles, with time spent in this stage around 10–25 minutes in the first cycle, and lengthening with each successive cycle.

Light sleep (Stages 1–2)

Time in Stage 1 before entering Stage 2 is around seven minutes. Time in Stage 2 is approximately 10–25 minutes in the first cycle, lengthening with each subsequent cycle.

Deep sleep (Stage 3)

Time in deep sleep is around 20–40 minutes in the first cycle but shortens with each subsequent cycle. It's common not to enter this stage after the second cycle.

Stages and cycles of sleep

A typical night of sleep will contain between 4–5 cycles, shown by the peaks and troughs on this graph. Each cycle is slightly different, with deeper sleep coming earlier in the night and more REM later on.

the brain is in a similarly active state to being awake. This is the stage during which memories and emotions are processed and dreams experienced.

Brain activity during each stage can be identified by its "signature" frequency measured in Hertz (Hz): "alpha" waves (8–13 Hz), characteristic of light Stage-1 sleep; "theta" waves (4–8 Hz) ,found during sleep Stages 1 and 2; and "delta" waves (up to 4 Hz), found in Stage-3 deep sleep. During REM sleep, both "beta" waves (13–30 Hz) and "theta" activity can be seen. Each sleep stage performs a different function, so it's important we experience enough of each to ensure that the processes they perform are completed. When this doesn't happen, we are left feeling lethargic and sleepy—known as sleep inertia.

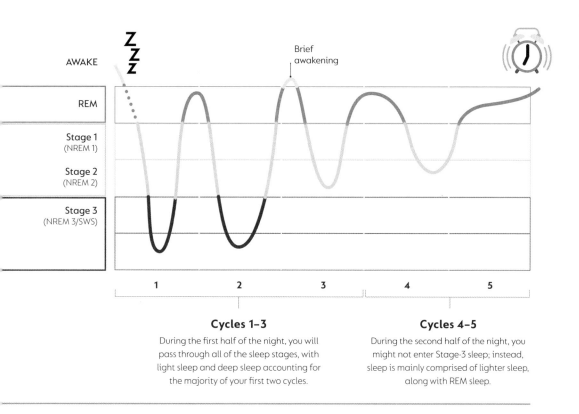

AWAKE

Brief awakening

REM

Stage 1 (NREM 1)

Stage 2 (NREM 2)

Stage 3 (NREM 3/SWS)

1   2   3   4   5

Cycles 1–3

During the first half of the night, you will pass through all of the sleep stages, with light sleep and deep sleep accounting for the majority of your first two cycles.

Cycles 4–5

During the second half of the night, you might not enter Stage-3 sleep; instead, sleep is mainly comprised of lighter sleep, along with REM sleep.

Dreaming

Sleep scientists are in agreement that to a greater or lesser extent, we all dream. As to the precise purpose and function of dreaming, there is no consensus—but research shows that when we do dream, much of the brain is still highly active.

Dreams are essentially a collection of thoughts and emotions unique to each person that usually (but not always) take place during REM sleep. For thousands of years, humans have sought to find meaning in their dreams, and there are many theories as to why we dream—from the idea that dreams are a stage on which we can rehearse social interaction or practice our responses to threatening situations, to the suggestion by the pioneer of psychoanalysis Sigmund Freud that they somehow represent our deepest wishes or unconscious, repressed desires.

Whether these theories hold any truth is still not clear, but there is an increasing body of scientific evidence that suggests dreaming might play an important role in the processing of memories and emotions, allowing us to "relive" certain events and feelings as we sleep in order to help the brain make sense of and store them as memories. REM sleep in particular seems to play a role in regulating our emotions, and as most of our dreams occur during the REM stage, this might also explain why our dreams are often vivid and super-charged with feelings.

When it comes to the question of whether dreaming is important for sleep itself, the fact that you dream at all is a strong indicator of REM sleep and a marker of good sleep—you can only reach the REM stage if sleep is uninterrupted. Another benefit for sleep quality is that dreaming has been shown to block out certain external noises, so it can play a role in helping you stay asleep.

Parietal cortex

Responsible for physical movement, this area of the brain is largely inactive during dreaming, which helpfully prevents us from acting out dreams.

Prefrontal cortex

The rational part of the brain is turned off, allowing dreams to be surreal, bizarre, and unconstrained by the rules of logic.

Visual cortex

The part of the brain responsible for what we see stays switched on and generates the vivid imagery we experience in dreams.

Hippocampus

The part of the brain involved in learning remains active, allowing fragments of memories to drop into our dreams, assisting with their consolidation.

The dreaming brain

With advances in measuring brain activity, scientists are now able to pinpoint the specific areas of the brain that are more active during the dream state. These discoveries may help unlock the mysteries of precisely how and why we dream.

Amygdala

The brain's center of emotions is extremely active during dreaming.

Good sleep, bad sleep

Aiming for perfect sleep every night is an unrealistic goal; we all have the odd bad night. When it comes to assessing whether the sleep you get is "good," it's just as much about quality as quantity.

Some lucky people never give their sleep a second thought, but for anyone struggling with their slumber, this is an almost unbelievable concept. For them, worrying about getting a "good" night's sleep is an ever-present concern.

So what exactly does good sleep look like? Sleep needs are as individual as your fingerprint; genetics, lifestyle, health conditions, and age all dictate the sleep you need to be at your best the following day. By far, the best benchmark of good sleep is how well-rested you feel when you wake up. After a good night's sleep, you should feel restored, alert, and ready to go. If this is you, then chances are you're getting good sleep— including enough Stage-3 sleep, which is where the majority of your brain and body's repair functions take place.

If you have difficulty falling asleep, problems staying asleep, or you often wake feeling tired and sluggish, it could be a sign of insomnia, but don't panic. From time to time, each of us will experience a bad night—it's completely normal. Remember: biologically, we know how to sleep. Many problems are temporary and have a simple solution, and some will resolve themselves without much intervention. Some sleep quirks, such as sleepwalking, are not a major cause for concern. Other issues such as teeth grinding are problems that can be rectified with appropriate treatment. However, there are a few issues that should always be followed up, as they may point to more serious conditions. Loud snoring or gasping for air in your sleep, sleep fragmentation (repeated interruptions during the night that lead to excessive tiredness during the day), or bouts of sleeplessness lasting more than four weeks will all require professional advice. A list of what a sleep specialist looks for when assessing the quality of your sleep is on the opposite page. Use this as a starting point to rate your sleep, but don't get too hung up on the results. This book will show you plenty of ways you can get the sleep you deserve if you're not quite there yet.

"Good sleep" assessment

Sleep clinicians assess the quality of a patient's sleep by applying various criteria. These can be broken down into the following four categories:

- **Sleep latency:** The time you take to fall asleep. You should ideally be asleep within 30 minutes of going to bed; if not, this suggests you aren't quite ready for sleep. Sleep trackers can be unreliable when it comes to measuring sleep latency; for instance, if you are reading a book, it may assess, from your lack of movement, that you are already asleep.

- **Time spent in different sleep phases:** On average, 50–60 percent of the night should be spent in light sleep, 13–23 percent in deep sleep, and 20–25 percent in REM. However, as you get older, you need less deep sleep. Spending the correct amount of time in each stage is more likely when you get a stretch of uninterrupted sleep.

- **Total sleep time:** Most adults need between 7–9 hours of sleep. This changes as you age (see pages 18–19), as does whether this amount is consecutive or a larger chunk of sleep supplemented with a nap. The key is how you feel the next day; the right amount and type of sleep for your personal needs should leave you feeling good when you wake.

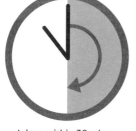

Asleep within 30 mins

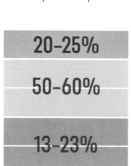

REM 20–25%

Light sleep 50–60%

Deep sleep 13–23%

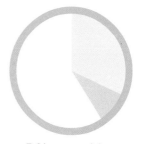

7–9 hours per night

- **Sleep efficiency:** This is the scoring a specialist will use to determine your quality of sleep. You can work yours out by dividing the amount of time spent asleep (in minutes) by the total amount of time in bed (in minutes), then multiplying this by 100. A sleep efficiency of 85 percent or higher suggests you are sleeping well, but slight fluctuations outside of this are normal.

Minutes spent asleep

Minutes spent in bed

$$\frac{\text{minutes asleep}}{\text{minutes in bed}} \times 100 = \textbf{sleep efficiency \%}$$

Forming good sleep habits

Many sleep specialists talk about the importance of "sleep hygiene"; put simply, this is a set of guidelines that will help maximize your chances of getting the best and most restful sleep.

4
Take care with caffeine
Caffeine lingers in your system and has a sleep-blocking effect (see pages 154–155). Try to avoid consuming caffeine after 2 p.m.

2
Keep a routine
The body thrives on consistency. Focus on a consistent sleep and wake time seven days a week.

1
Prioritize sleep
Work out how much sleep you need (see pages 18–19) and count back from the time you need to get up to figure out when to go to bed to ensure you get this.

5
Avoid nicotine and alcohol
Nicotine is a stimulant and promotes alertness (see page 159). Alcohol is a sedative but disrupts sleep (see page 157).

3
Get enough natural light
Heading outside early in the morning and keeping lights low at night helps synchronize your circadian rhythm.

6
Reduce stimulation
Avoid social media and emails at night. Think about your TV choices; an action movie is more likely to overstimulate you and keep you awake and alert.

A good routine

"Sleep hygiene" sounds cold and clinical, but it's simply a description of the ways in which you can make it easier to get into the habit of great sleep. Use this list as a stepping-off point for forming your own routine rather than as a rigid prescription.

The quality of your sleep depends on many factors—which are covered in this book—but developing positive habits is a great place to start in your quest for better sleep. However, it's worth remembering that the healthiest habit of all is to relax. Worrying about achieving the "perfect" conditions for sleep can be counterproductive, so look at building sleep hygiene into your life as an act of self-care—a way to wind down and create an environment that gives you the best chance of sleeping well.

7
Comfort is key
Sleep is an all-around sensory process, so ensure that the room is cool and that your bed, bedding, and nightclothes are all comfortable.

10
Relax
Stress is linked to sleep problems. Develop relaxation practices that you enjoy and do them regularly (see pages 80–81).

8
Be active
Exercise helps regulate your circadian rhythm. Think about when to exercise to leave yourself enough time for winding and cooling down before bed (see pages 82–83).

12
Cut the noise
Sudden noises wake most people, but ongoing noise can reduce sleep quality. Consider earplugs or sound-masking devices (see pages 188–189).

11
Create a safe haven
Make your bedroom into a sleep sanctuary—somewhere you actively want to be and find enticing (see pages 170–171).

9
Take daytime naps
To boost energy, set the alarm for 30 mins and close your eyes. Avoid longer naps—this could mean you wake from deep sleep and feel groggy, not refreshed (see pages 138–139).

Keeping a sleep journal

A sleep journal doesn't just record when you sleep, it tracks everything you do over a 24-hour period. It can help you get to know your own sleep and build a picture of how your sleep affects your day and vice versa.

By regularly keeping track of things such as what time you wake; when you eat, exercise, and smoke; intake of caffeine and alcohol; the activities you do around bedtime; when you go to bed; and if you wake in the night, you can start to see patterns and assess if any of these are playing a role in your quality and quantity of sleep.

To get to the heart of what shapes your sleep, you can also use your sleep journal to record your mood and energy levels across the day and to note how long it took you to fall asleep after getting into bed.

Should you be referred to a sleep clinic, your sleep journal is a key tool in helping clinicians diagnose any issues. The data you provide will be used to calculate your sleep efficiency (see pages 32–33). This will be a useful starting point for setting measurable goals for sleep improvement.

To track your sleep at home, use the journal on the opposite page for around two weeks. You don't have to be super-accurate about times—anxious clock watching will only worsen any sleep worries you have. Simply fill it out when you wake in the morning and again at various points throughout the day. After two weeks, you can start to look for patterns. Is your sleep worse after a stressful day at work? Do you sleep better after an evening bath? Or if you take some downtime before heading to bed? Once you identify what might be getting in the way of sleep, you can take steps to address these factors.

Tracking sleep and what influences it
By logging activities such as when you drink coffee and exercise, you can find out if they affect your sleep. These are only some suggestions to note—be sure to capture information personal to you.

☐ Awake
⬤ In bed but awake
◼ Asleep
○ Wake in the night
⊠ Naps

You can use these timings to work out your sleep efficiency: minutes asleep divided by minutes in bed x 100

A visual guide to your sleep may help you create a picture of your sleep pattern

Tuesday January 12th

| 6 p.m. | 12 midnight | 6 a.m. | 12 noon | 6 p.m. |

1. What time did you get into bed? — *10:35 p.m.*

2. What time did you try to go to sleep? — *11:30 p.m.*

3. How long did it take you to fall asleep? — *30 mins*

4. How many times did you wake up, not counting your final awakening? — *3 times*

5. In total, how long did these awakenings last? — *1 hour 10 mins*

6. What time was your final awakening? — *7:35 a.m.*

7. What time did you get out of bed for the day? — *8:20 a.m.*

8. Did you take a nap? At what time and for how long? — *2:30 p.m. for 20 mins*

9. How would you rate the quality of your sleep?

   ☐ Very poor   ☐ Poor   ☑ Fair   ☐ Good   ☐ Very good

Other comments

- *4 beers at 9 p.m.*
- *Coffee at 10 a.m. and 4 p.m.*
- *Went for a run at 8 a.m.*
- *Worried about big presentation at work*

Your mood can affect your perception of sleep

The time of day you exercise can help or hinder sleep

Both alcohol and caffeine affect sleep

Both stress and worry can affect sleep

How long you nap can affect how you feel for the rest of the day and nighttime sleep

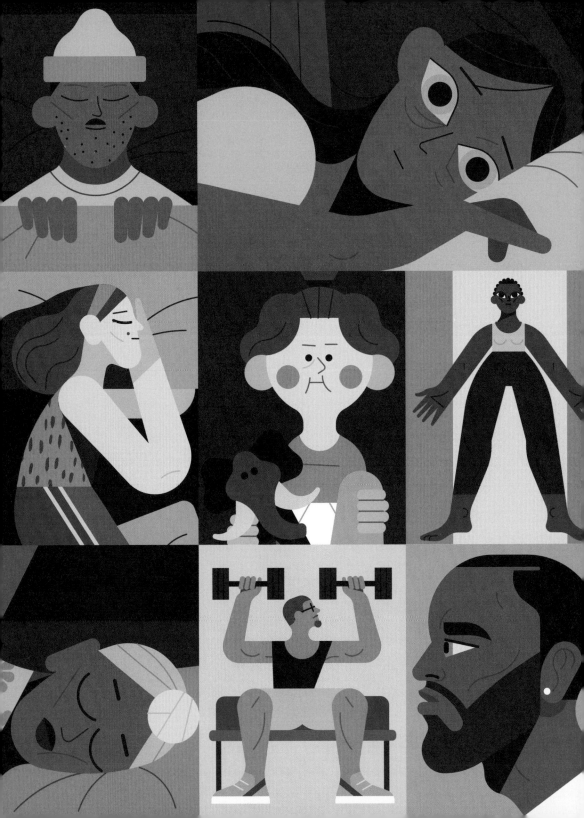

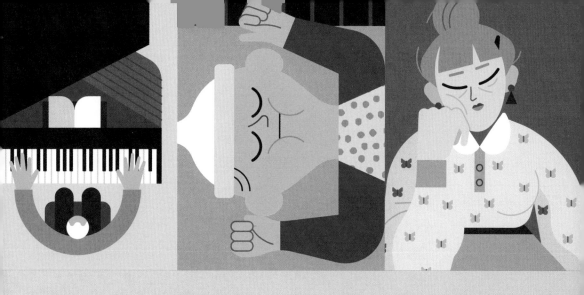

KNOW YOUR OWN SLEEP

Many factors may affect your sleep for better or worse: the job you do, your eating and exercise habits, underlying health issues, even the person (or pet) you share a bed with. Understanding your personal sleep profile is key.

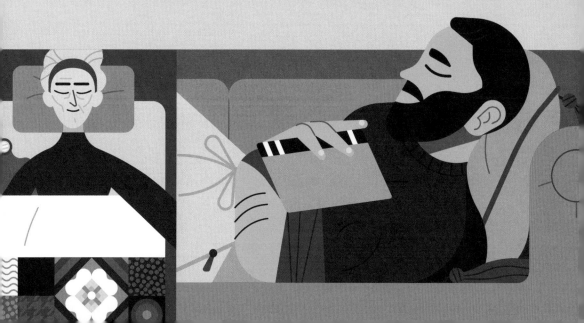

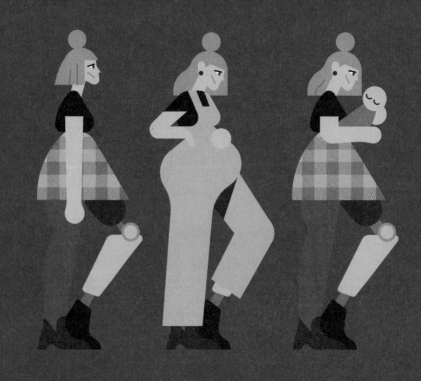

Life stages

As our bodies and circumstances change
throughout our lives, so too do our sleep needs.
Each milestone brings potential challenges to
achieving the sleep you need, but by arming
yourself with the right knowledge and
strategies, you can overcome issues or prevent
them from arising in the first place.

Should I sleep train my baby?

"Sleep training" is a term that covers a wide range of gentle techniques designed to help your baby learn to sleep independently.

There are many reasons for wanting to encourage your baby to sleep on a schedule. From the baby's perspective, learning to self-soothe, settle themselves to sleep, and develop a consistent sleep pattern is key for development and well-being. As for you, the evidence is clear: you need enough good sleep to function well in your caring role.

A newborn's circadian rhythm takes three or four months to develop, and their melatonin levels are relatively low. Establishing a sleeping pattern during this time is biologically difficult and probably pointless—leave it until your baby reaches at least the three-month mark.

The topic of sleep training and bedtime routines is an emotional one for many parents. Studies of methods have not been conclusive, due partly to the difficulty in conducting a large enough study, and differences in

TEARS AND FEARS

Crying can be upsetting to witness, but it's perfectly normal. One study showed that following a short period of crying at bedtime, babies' cortisol (stress) levels on waking were not raised. Also, follow-up assessments showed that the relationship between parent and child was unaffected.

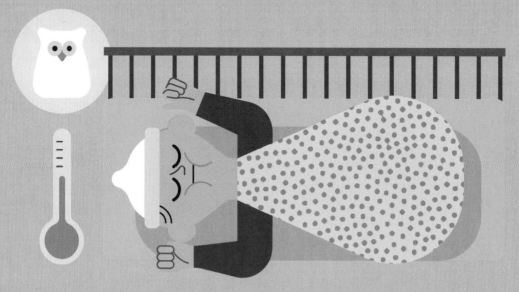

subjective reports of parents as to how their baby slept. Whatever you decide to do, it's a personal choice, and as with all sleep issues, there is no one-size-fits-all solution. Teething, growth spurts, and changes in environment are all normal disruptors of any baby's sleep routine—and as they grow, their sleep patterns will inevitably change. Nothing lasts forever—not even your baby's sleepless nights!

WINDING DOWN FOR BEDTIME

Whether or not you wish to sleep train, all babies (and their carers!) will benefit from creating a soothing, sleep-inducing environment.

• **Put your baby to bed drowsy** rather than already asleep. If they wake in new surroundings, it can be harder for them to go back to sleep on their own.

• **Keep room temperature** at 64–68°F (18–20°C), as being too hot can prevent the baby from falling asleep. Try a lightweight sleep sack so they are covered all night and less likely to wake due to getting cold.

• **Reduce light in the evening**, as too much light can delay sleepiness. For feedings and so on during the night, use a plug-in, low-level red light in the baby's room—red light is proven to be less disruptive to sleep patterns.

• **Wake your baby** at the same time every morning, regardless of a late bedtime or disturbed night. This helps build the baby's sleep pressure through the day, making sleep easier the following night.

SLEEP TRAINING TECHNIQUES

Graduated extinction/ Ferber method

Put your baby to bed drowsy and after one minute, leave the room. Then return and stroke or speak to them, but don't pick them up. Gradually increase the length of your absences until your baby can fall asleep alone.

Camping out

Put your baby down to sleep and sit near them until they doze off, then leave the room. Each night, move a little farther away toward the door. Eventually, your baby learns to get to sleep without you in the room.

Bedtime fading

To encourage your baby's internal clock to align to an earlier bedtime, you gradually, over days or weeks, shift bedtime in 15-minute increments. If they don't settle, soothe them as normal.

Cry it out (extinction method)

Similar to the Ferber method, but after putting the baby to bed, you leave them to cry if they don't settle. This controversial method is simply too distressing for both babies and parents and is not recommended.

How can I soothe an overtired baby to sleep?

At bedtime after a busy day, your baby won't settle and is getting increasingly upset. They have passed the point of drowsiness, and despite seeming exhausted an hour ago, sleep is now out of the question.

Following a hectic or stimulating day, an overtired baby can experience sensory overload in response. This overwhelms their sympathetic nervous system (see pages 208–209), triggering a surge of stress hormones adrenaline and cortisol, which override sleepiness. A simple way to help put this process into reverse is by rocking.

ROCKABYE BABY

A baby in the womb is constantly rocked, and this sets up a primary association between the motion and feeling secure. In their first year, your baby will continue to be rocked—in your arms or in a sling, rocker, stroller, or car. In this way, rocking becomes naturally associated with sleep.

Research has found that rocking triggers a set of cardiac and motor responses in the baby's body and brain that have a significantly calming effect. It also activates the baby's sense of awareness of their own body—known as proprioception (see page 177). And it's not only babies who benefit—one study in adults found that a rocking motion caused people to fall asleep more quickly and enjoy more restorative, slow-wave sleep.

If your baby is overtired, it's important to calm them before you start any part of their bedtime routine. It may take longer, but this helps prevent the baby from forming negative associations with bedtime. Ultimately, it's essential to ensure that the baby links rocking with being soothed rather than being persuaded to sleep; otherwise, they may learn to rely on rocking to be able to fall asleep.

Studies of crying babies show that their heart rate

slows

much more rapidly if the baby is picked up and carried, compared to being held by someone who is sitting down

How do I help a toddler sleep through the night?

Toddlers are active, curious beings who constantly want to explore—which can make getting them to fall asleep and stay asleep challenging.

Young children between the ages of 1 and 2 become more aware of their surroundings and want to discover all that the world has to offer them. This, along with constantly developing physical, cognitive, social, and motor skills, means that helping them sleep through the night can be tricky. Every child is unique, but following some key sleep-promoting strategies can help:

- **Consistency is key** Regular bed and wake times will help your toddler's body "know" when it's time for sleep. A pleasurable but low-key set routine provides your child with a sense of predictability and security around bedtime.

- **Use a night light and timer** This helps train your toddler's brain to make the association—when the light goes off and it's dark, it's time to sleep. There is some evidence that a red light enhances sleep quality and improves alertness on waking.

- **Avoid late naps** A toddler needs around five hours of wakefulness to build enough sleep pressure to be tired at night, so if bedtime is 7 p.m., try to ensure there are no more naps after 2 p.m.

- **Low stimulation** Bedrooms are often full of toys, and the temptation to climb out of bed and play can be overwhelming. Put toys out of sight to create a distraction-free sleep environment.

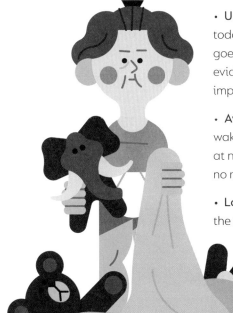

Can lack of sleep affect growth?

The secretion of human growth hormone peaks during deep sleep, so a pattern of poor sleeping can have an effect on this vital body chemical.

Human growth hormone is essential for overall growth in children, and in adults it maintains strength and regulates metabolism. For both children and adults, it is necessary for cell repair—particularly when recovering from exercise, injury, or illness. Growth hormone is released by the pituitary gland throughout the day, but peak levels are secreted during the deeper stages of sleep—so a lack of good sleep will reduce the overall amount of the hormone in your body.

Happily, poor sleep will have little effect on children's growth, because the resulting hormone shortfall is compensated for by the huge surges that occur during a child's growth spurts.

For adults, however, losing out on hormone production due to poor sleep is more of an issue. It can lead to reduced muscle mass and strength, thinning hair, and weaker bones. Although other factors may be at play, ensuring you get enough deep sleep will boost your body's natural growth and repair functions.

Growth hormone release

This hormone is released throughout the day, but certain activities, such as eating or exercise, cause it to spike. The biggest peak occurs during deep sleep.

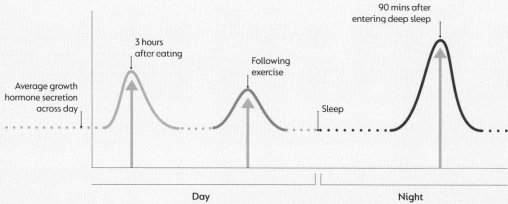

90 mins after entering deep sleep

3 hours after eating

Following exercise

Average growth hormone secretion across day

Sleep

Day

Night

Will my child grow out of night terrors?

Any parent who has witnessed their child experiencing a night terror will testify to how distressing it can be. Night terrors are brief episodes, usually lasting up to 15 minutes, where your child might scream, sweat, appear terrified, and move around before abruptly falling back asleep. Different from nightmares, which happen during REM sleep and can be remembered, night terrors usually occur in the early part of the night during deep, non-REM sleep. They are not technically dreams, but a sudden fear reaction driven by the fight-or-flight stress response and resulting spike in adrenaline.

Despite often having their eyes open, your child is not fully awake and will not recognize you during an episode. Because of this, waking your child from this state to comfort them can leave them more disoriented and confused, and they will take longer to settle back down.

NO CAUSE FOR ALARM

Episodes can be triggered by stress, tiredness, a change in sleep schedule, medication, or a fever and are more likely to occur in girls than boys. Studies in twins suggest a genetic component, and there is also a link with sleepwalking—research shows that a child of two parents who are, or were, sleepwalkers is more likely to experience night terrors, and around one-third of children who have terrors develop sleepwalking as they grow older.

No matter how alarming a night terror may be for you as a parent, rest assured that they won't do your child any lasting physical or psychological harm—children rarely remember episodes. The most common age for children to experience night terrors is 2–4 years, but they can continue until age 12; reassuringly, most children grow out of them by the time they reach their teens.

HOW TO HELP

In some children, night terrors happen at roughly the same time each night, so it can help to gently wake your child shortly before an anticipated episode. Because they have been in a deep sleep, they will likely fall asleep again very quickly. Try doing this for seven consecutive nights; this can be enough to break the pattern without affecting their overall sleep quality.

Does the school day fit in with my teenager's sleep needs?

Anyone with a teenager will testify to the daily struggle of waking them up for school, but is this sleepy stupor and inability to focus in the mornings simply a matter of teenage laziness, or something more?

During puberty, not only are teens experiencing a hormonal storm, but they may also be suffering from chronic sleep deprivation. It's not that teens are inherently lazy; their tendency to drift off in midmorning classes is partly down to them being denied their natural sleeping routine, which differs from that of children and adults.

BODY CLOCK SHIFT

When puberty hits, the circadian rhythm (see pages 22–23) jumps forward by around two hours, likely due to growth- and sex-hormone surges, so production of melatonin (the sleepiness hormone) occurs later in the day. This means that expecting a teen to sleep at 11 p.m. is like an adult being sent to bed at 8 p.m. And for teens, rising at 7 a.m. is as painful as if an adult were hauled out of bed at 4 a.m.

Because they are not yet ready for sleep, many teens hang out online late into the night, further stimulating their brain and keeping them awake. This leads to "social jet lag," with teens getting less sleep on school days and sleeping longer on weekends, making them even less able to meet the demands of their school day.

A later school start and finish time would benefit teens, and of the schools that have tried this, all report improved grades and student engagement, as well as a drop in lateness and absences. Getting your teen's school to try this might not be possible, but you can help lessen daytime sleepiness—see opposite page. When teens reach adulthood, the biological clock shifts back and this built-in time lag gradually recedes.

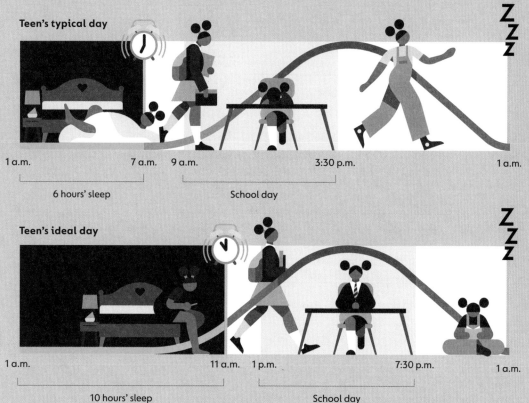

Teen's typical day

1 a.m. 7 a.m. 9 a.m. 3:30 p.m. 1 a.m.

6 hours' sleep School day

Teen's ideal day

1 a.m. 11 a.m. 1 p.m. 7:30 p.m. 1 a.m.

10 hours' sleep School day

KEY

- Sleeping
- Groggy
- Semi-alert
- Fully alert

Sleep later, learn better

Each graph charts a teen's daily alertness levels. A later school start means they are alert for the whole school day, but on a typical schedule, their alertness peaks just as school ends.

SUPPORTING A SLEEPY TEEN

- **For younger teens, keep digital devices** out of their room at night. If they are older, turning off the household WiFi at a set time each night shows you are willing to stick to the rules, too! Suggest alternative evening activities like reading or listening to a podcast, which are relaxing and help keep sleep-inhibiting levels of the stress hormone cortisol down.

- **Exposure to bright light in the morning** and low light at night can help shift your teen's sleep schedule back, so consider a dimmer on their bedroom light, or try using an orange or red bulb in their bedside lamp.

49

How much does screen time affect my teenager's sleep?

Technology use is on the rise among all age groups, but particularly among teenagers. So how concerned should parents be about the impact of digital devices on their children's ability to sleep?

Digital devices are now commonplace in the bedroom, and sleep issues in teens are rising, so it seems logical to make a connection between the two.

However, a recent study found that children's sleep is not significantly affected by screen time, with only a few minutes lost for every hour of screen use as measured throughout the day.

So if it's not the amount of time spent on the screens themselves, could it be how and when teens are using screens that causes their sleep problems? Using digital devices in the evening, when natural sleepiness should kick in, means the urge to sleep is overridden by the excitement of what's happening on screen, and this stimulation seems to be a factor in making teens more awake.

Perhaps the answer lies in simply telling teens to turn their screens off at a reasonable time, but anyone who has tried this will know it often leads to arguments. Teens' body clocks run later than their parents' (see pages 48–49), and the urge to stay up late socializing online can feel irresistible. Most teens live a huge portion of their lives online, and many struggle with FOMO—a fear of missing out—when they aren't online and interacting with friends.

To help teens get better sleep, encourage them to get enough natural light and exercise during the day; both dramatically improve sleep (see pages 34–35). Also try being open to hearing about their worries—this way, you can help them manage these—and accept that a calm, consistent evening routine is a more effective antidote to FOMO than taking the smartphone to bed.

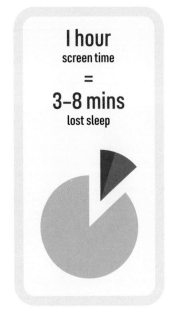

1 hour
screen time
=
3–8 mins
lost sleep

" " _____

FOMO—the fear of
missing out—is stressful
for many teens and often
plays a significant role in
their sleep problems.

Why does my teen randomly seem to doze off in the daytime?

Having a constantly sleepy teen is pretty normal, but when there's enough stimulation to keep them awake and they still fall asleep, this may be a warning sign of something more serious.

Narcolepsy is a sudden and temporary loss of consciousness that can develop at any age, but usually appears in adolescence, with more than half of sufferers reporting their first symptoms as a teen.

Symptoms of this rare condition—it affects around 1 in 2,500 people—include fragmented sleep at night due to repeated waking. The next day, this results in excessive daytime sleepiness (EDS), leaving the sufferer likely to nod off at random times. During narcoleptic episodes, the sleeper quickly enters REM as they fall asleep and often experiences visual hallucinations.

Some people with narcolepsy may also experience a related, more dramatic condition called cataplexy—an abrupt loss of muscle control that causes them to collapse. Although a person experiencing cataplexy may appear unconscious, they are awake but temporarily paralyzed. Cataplexy is usually triggered by strong, positive emotions and associated behaviors, such as laughing, so it can be particularly distressing when it occurs during what should be an enjoyable experience or activity.

WHAT CAUSES NARCOLEPSY?

Research shows that narcolepsy may be linked to a lack of hypocretins (also called orexins), the neurotransmitters involved in the regulation of the normal sleep/wake cycle. This deficiency appears to cause the sleep/wake "switch" to flip on and off during the day. Research is ongoing, but factors such as age, genetics, and certain infections and illnesses all seem to play a part in triggering the condition.

SEEK HELP

If you suspect your teen might be suffering from narcolepsy, it's essential to seek support from your doctor. Narcolepsy is a lifelong condition that can be well managed with the right medication and good sleep hygiene (see pages 34–35).

How can I help my teen sleep better at test time?

Teenagers and tests can be a toxic combination: anxieties around performance coupled with disruption to their body clock can all lead to sleep deprivation.

We know that a teen's circadian rhythm shifts forward during adolescence (see pages 18–19), meaning they don't feel sleepy until later in the evening and need to sleep longer into the morning. A rigid timetable of tests makes no allowance for this, making it impossible for them to get enough sleep for effective learning and memory consolidation. That's why staying up all night to cram for a test is counterproductive and likely to lead to a cycle of sleep deprivation and sleep debt.

At test times, it's more important than ever to encourage your teen to stick to healthy sleep hygiene habits (see pages 34–35). They can also benefit from your help to set up a study routine. A daytime nap between study periods will help counter the sleep debt from all those early wake-ups on test days.

Nap-assisted learning

By studying in the morning, napping, then working again in the afternoon and evening, teens will get the sleep they need to alleviate the effects of an early wake-up call on test day. A long nap plus six hours of sleep at night will result in seven and a half hours of sleep overall.

KEY

Awake/resting
Study time
Sleep time

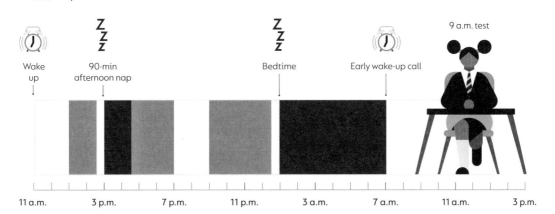

Wake up | 90-min afternoon nap | Bedtime | Early wake-up call | 9 a.m. test

11 a.m. 3 p.m. 7 p.m. 11 p.m. 3 a.m. 7 a.m. 11 a.m. 3 p.m.

Does sleep affect our ability to learn?

The brain needs sleep in order to effectively process and store information it has acquired throughout the day. During sleep, it actively consolidates and creates memories to be retrieved in the future.

Sleep helps you both remember and forget: while you sleep, the brain sifts through everything you have heard and seen that day, storing only those memories it considers to be useful or important. It's as if once you drop off, an army of filing clerks gets to work, moving what you need to remember from short-term to long-term memory, then ditching the rest.

SLEEP CONSOLIDATES MEMORY

Research into sleep and learning indicates that the declarative memory, which stores facts and events, is reinforced by slow-wave sleep, which you get more of in the first half of the night. Procedural memory, which helps us perform tasks without having to think about them (such as riding a bike), however, is consolidated by REM sleep, most of which happens later in the night.

Interestingly, recent research has also highlighted the importance of sleep spindles, bursts of brain activity that occur in Stage-2 sleep, in transferring memories into long-term storage. The length of time we spend in Stage-2 sleep increases over the course of the night, so this may be another reason why the overall length of your sleep affects learning ability.

Exactly how sleep aids learning is a complex area that needs further research, but given that different stages of sleep seem to facilitate different types of memory, ensuring that you get enough sleep to cycle through all the stages is an excellent way to help embed learning and memories.

SLEEP AND FORGETTING

As we age, the quality of slow-wave sleep decreases, and this appears to have a direct connection to brain deterioration and memory loss. Research is ongoing into whether good sleep can help protect against dementia and Alzheimer's (see pages 206–207).

Declarative memory
Facts and events, such as
birthdays and addresses

Procedural memory
Tasks, such as riding a bike or
learning a new language

Short-term memory formed
Hippocampus then "decides" which
memories need to be stored longer term

Consolidated by
slow-wave sleep

Consolidated by
REM sleep

Making memories

When we sleep, our brain
assesses everything we
have learned that day and
decides whether or not to
transfer it to our long-term
memory—from where it
can later be retrieved
and recalled.

**File in
long-term memory**

Trash

TIPS TO BOOST LEARNING

• Go to sleep within three
hours of learning something
new—studies have shown
that this improves memory
retention.

• When you wake up, review
what you've learned the day
before. This reactivates
the memory and helps
consolidate new information.

• Prioritize sleep. Studies
have shown that getting
more than six hours of sleep
at night boosts memory and
alertness by 25 percent.

How will being pregnant affect my sleep?

Each stage of pregnancy brings its own sleep challenges—so finding ways to get good-quality rest is vital. During pregnancy, you need more sleep to support your body as it works hard to promote your baby's growth and development, but the changes in your body can make getting good sleep more of a challenge.

FIRST TRIMESTER (WEEKS 1–12)

In your first three months, high levels of estrogen, progesterone, and human chorionic gonadotropin—the hormones that surge in order to maintain a pregnancy—have a warming effect on the body. They can also make you sleepier than usual. Increased estrogen may cause breast tenderness, and morning sickness (which isn't restricted to the morning!) can also disrupt sleep. During this trimester, trying not to overheat is the priority. Keep your bedroom cool and use light bedding and nightclothes. A cotton bra with loose support can help reduce the discomfort of tender breasts as you shift positions in bed.

SECOND TRIMESTER (WEEKS 13–28)

Insomnia can be an issue, as well as snoring and sleep apnea, which may be triggered by weight gain and raised estrogen levels. As the baby grows, it starts to squash up your body's organs, which can lead to heartburn and more frequent trips to the bathroom. Once the baby starts to move, a kick to your ribs in the night will definitely wake you up! Sleeping on your left side can minimize heartburn and snoring, and also boosts blood circulation, helping nutrients reach the placenta. If you have trouble getting to sleep, lavender essential oil has clinically proven sleep-inducing qualities. Use in a room diffuser or mix a few drops with water and spray your pillow before bed.

TAKE A NAP

If possible, grab every opportunity for a nap when you're pregnant. As your nighttime sleep may be more fractured, catching up during the day will help you feel rested and more energetic. Research also shows that napping may offer effective protection from developing chronic sleep issues in pregnancy.

THIRD TRIMESTER (WEEKS 29–40)

The final trimester is likely to be when your sleep is most disrupted. Your radically changed body shape means that backache, heartburn, restless legs, and swollen ankles may develop. As your bladder is compressed further, frequent bathroom visits are inevitable. Extra pillows or cushions will offer support as you try to find a comfortable position. "Pregnancy pillows" are extra long and designed to support the whole length of the body—many people find them helpful in the later stages. Most of the issues causing poor sleep will disappear once the baby is born, but if you continue to experience symptoms such as restless legs, insomnia, or snoring, seek your doctor's advice.

Optimal sleep positions

As your bump grows, it's most likely that sleeping on your side will be most comfortable. A pillow between your legs helps keep the spine aligned, avoiding back pain.

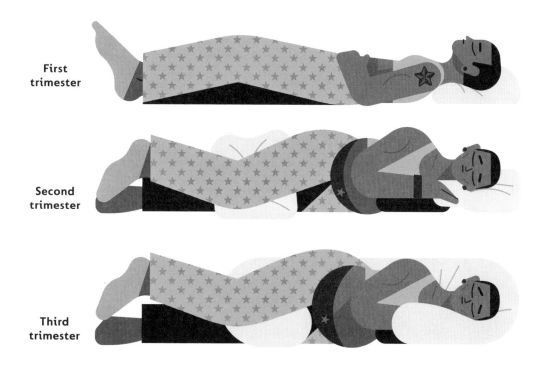

First trimester

Second trimester

Third trimester

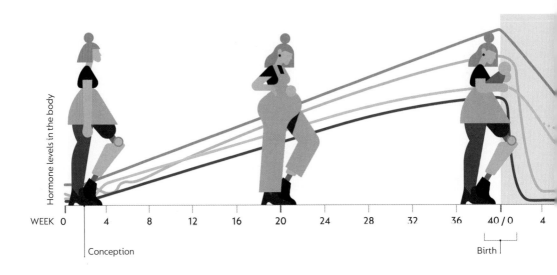

Hormone levels in the body

WEEK 0   4   8   12   16   20   24   28   32   36   40 / 0   4

Conception   Birth

I'm a new parent. Will lack of sleep wreck my health?

A new baby often means that your regular sleep patterns are disrupted, if not destroyed, and this can take a huge physical and mental toll on sleep-deprived carers.

If you've just given birth, your hormones are in a state of chaos; this, as well as getting up every few hours to feed your baby, can severely impact quantity and quality of sleep. Sex hormones estrogen and progesterone improve sleep quality and reduce the time it takes to get to sleep, and levels of these drop drastically after you give birth and can take several weeks to return to normal. Stress hormone cortisol, which helps regulate the sleep/wake cycle, also drops after birth, and this can disrupt natural sleep patterns. However, as hormone levels gradually even out, your ability to sleep will usually improve.

It's normal for new parents to feel exhausted but, reassuringly, there's no data to indicate that sleep deficits in early parenthood lead to any long-term health

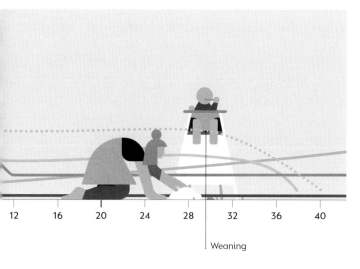

12   16   20   24   28   32   36   40

| Weaning

Hormones during and after pregnancy

Levels of sex and stress hormones rise during pregnancy until the point of birth, when they dip drastically—except for prolactin, which tapers off gradually if breastfeeding. By about eight weeks postbirth, hormones should return to prepregnancy levels, and periods resume their usual fluctuating cycles (see page 90).

KEY

- Cortisol
- Estrogen
- Progesterone
- Prolactin—breastfeeding
- Prolactin—nonbreastfeeding

problems. To help yourself through this temporary torture, try these techniques:

- **Catch a nap** whenever your baby does. Napping gives a burst of Stage-2 sleep that improves alertness and mood.

- **If you are coparenting**, alternate "night duties" so each of you regularly gets an undisturbed night's sleep.

- **Keep the lights low** during night feeds to help you get back to sleep more easily.

- **Don't rely on coffee** and sugary snacks to keep you going. These disrupt your body clock further and can disturb sleep when you finally do go to bed.

- **Try to stick to your regular bedtime** and wake-up time, even after a particularly disrupted night. This helps your body clock stay on track.

BREASTFEEDING AND SLEEP

During pregnancy, prolactin—the hormone responsible for milk production—increases up to twenty-fold, and if you are breastfeeding, these levels remain high. Prolactin can also promote REM sleep, and some studies have indicated that breastfeeding may help mothers sleep. However, prolactin isn't a significant enough sleep enhancer to make it a major factor in deciding whether to breastfeed or for how long.

Menopause is causing havoc with my sleep: what can I do?

Among the challenges women face around menopause, disrupted sleep can be a major one, with around 65 percent of women reporting issues—but there are ways to manage this impact.

Menopause, when the monthly menstrual cycle stops, is usually divided into phases that describe the different stages of hormonal change. The biological changes that take place at each stage can lead to significant sleep issues—and some of the other common symptoms of menopause can compound this problem.

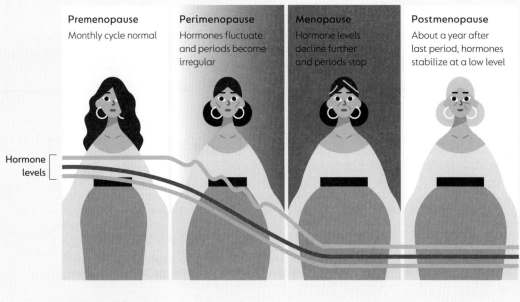

Premenopause
Monthly cycle normal

Perimenopause
Hormones fluctuate and periods become irregular

Menopause
Hormone levels decline further and periods stop

Postmenopause
About a year after last period, hormones stabilize at a low level

Hormone levels

Hormonal changes
As menopause approaches, hormone production starts to fluctuate and fall, triggering a variety of symptoms.

KEY

- Estrogen
- Progesterone
- Melatonin

HOW MENOPAUSE AFFECTS SLEEP

During perimenopause, the phase leading up to periods stopping, production of estrogen and progesterone, the two main sex hormones, declines. Fluctuating levels of estrogen can lead to night sweats and hot flashes, and a drop in progesterone can also cause anxiety, depression, and weight gain, all of which can interfere with sleep. The sleep hormone melatonin also declines, influenced both by age and by decreasing estrogen and progesterone. This can leave many people either unable to fall or stay asleep or waking too early to feel rested.

Hot flashes are one of the most sleep-disruptive menopausal symptoms, causing a sudden feeling of heat that spreads over the body, leading to sweating, increased heart rate, and flushed skin. They usually last a few minutes, but can linger for 20 minutes or more. Keeping cool is key to preventing hot flashes from waking you up or hindering your ability to get to sleep in the first place.

REPLACING THE HORMONES

Hormone replacement therapy (HRT) has proved effective in treating sleep disruption during the menopause. Different types of HRT consist of estrogen, progesterone, or a combination of the two. Replacing estrogen can stop or reduce the frequency of hot flashes; progesterone may improve slow-wave sleep and can also help counteract weight gain that can cause other sleep issues. Talk to your doctor to decide if HRT is right for you. Consider also psychological support such as counseling, which can be very helpful if your sleep is affected by anxiety or low mood associated with menopause.

MANAGING NIGHT-TIME HOT FLASHES

• Keep spare nightwear next to your bed so you can change out of sweaty clothes and get back to sleep more quickly.

• If you share a bed, a cooling mattress pad on your side can help, as can covers with different tog ratings.

• Try cutting back on or avoiding known triggers, such as caffeine and alcohol.

• Eating foods rich in hormone-balancing phytoestrogens, such as tofu and chickpeas, can help prevent episodes.

• Take an omega-3 supplement, or eat plenty of omega-3-rich oily fish or flaxseeds.

Why is it the older I get, the worse I sleep?

It's completely normal for the body's sleep needs to naturally change across your lifetime, but it's the shift in circadian rhythms, plus other physical changes, that can cause disrupted sleep for older people.

In later life, you require fewer growth and cell-repair functions, so the amount of sleep you need does decrease slightly, although not as much as many of us assume (see pages 18–19). The requirement of good sleep for good health remains, but many older people report a worse quality of sleep than when they were younger and are often sleep-deprived.

OUT OF SYNC

As we age, less exposure to natural light (possibly due to spending more time indoors), plus a natural decline in melatonin production, can mean we are short on the natural cues that tell us when to sleep and wake. This can have a detrimental effect on our ability to regulate our sleep pattern.

Sleep well as you age

1
See the light
Get lots of daylight every day. If this is a problem for you, fit light bulbs that mimic daylight—look for those in the 5,000–6,500K range.

2
Nap if you need to
Take a nap in the afternoon to boost energy. Keep it short—20–30 minutes—or you may disrupt the following night's sleep.

Some of the issues that can come with age—such as decreased bone density and stiffer joints—may mean it's harder to get and stay comfortable in bed. As we age, the metabolism slows down, which for some can mean an increase in weight. If weight gain is significant, it can lead to snoring or obstructive sleep apnea—both of which can disrupt sleep.

Another factor is the need to visit the bathroom more often. For men, lower testosterone or an enlarged prostate gland can both cause more frequent urination. For women, the trigger for this change in habits is often the disruption to hormones during and after menopause.

Any of these factors, added to the fact that levels of deep sleep naturally decline with age, can lead to less time in deep sleep, so that you end up not getting the rest you need—and making a minor sleep issue worse. There is a perception that poor sleep is a given as you age, but this definitely need not be the case. Try the simple strategies below and you will likely see your sleep improve.

THE EFFECTS OF MEDICATION

As we get older, it becomes more likely that we'll be prescribed medication for health issues that arise. With any new medication, it's worth checking with a doctor or pharmacist whether its side effects include changes to sleep. Beta blockers, for example, which are commonly prescribed for high blood pressure, can reduce the body's ability to produce melatonin and impact sleep patterns as a result.

3
Keep it regular
Even if you no longer need to get up for work, sticking to a consistent routine of sleep and wake times keeps your circadian rhythm on track.

4
Get moving
Keeping mobile helps to lubricate joints and maintain a healthy weight. Yoga and walking both boost the body's systems and promote sleep.

5
Avoid nightcaps
If you can, don't have any drinks in the two or three hours before bed. This will reduce nighttime bathroom visits and mean less sleep disruption.

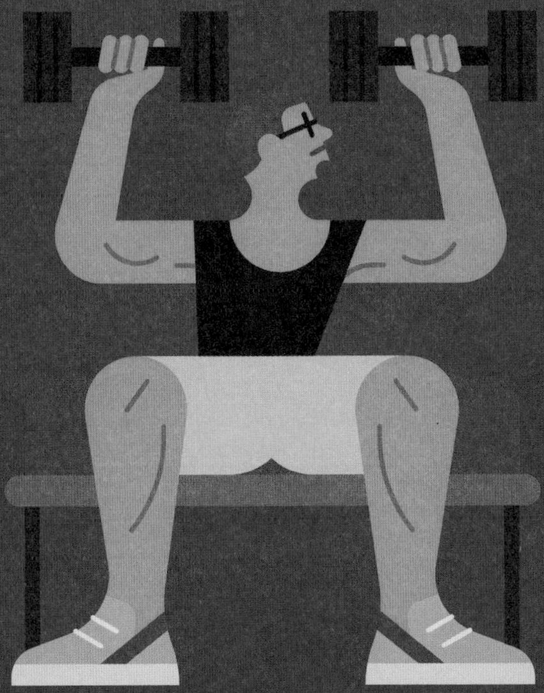

Mind and body

The mind and body have a two-way
relationship with sleep: our mental and
physical health can affect how we sleep, and
the quality and quantity of our sleep can also
have a significant effect on our sense of
well-being and long-term health.

Why do we yawn?

Scientists have reached little agreement about why we yawn. The average adult yawns around 20 times per day. Surely this universal reflex serves some purpose? Humans do it, animals do it, even babies in the womb do it. But explaining why we yawn is tricky—there are many theories but little evidence to back most of them up.

One popular theory is that we yawn due to boredom. When bored, energy is low and we don't breathe as deeply; low oxygen levels in the body therefore trigger a yawn in order to replenish our supply. Another idea is that the increased intake of air cools the brain. When we don't get enough sleep, brain temperature increases, and this explains why we yawn when we are tired.

Yet another interesting suggestion is that yawning helps alleviate the feeling that you can't breathe, which is common during times of stress and anxiety. Yawning helps by expanding the rib cage, sending a signal to the brain that the body has taken in sufficient oxygen.

" "
Reading this might make you yawn—just thinking about yawning triggers a yawn in 88% of people.

PSYCHOPATHS DON'T YAWN

Contagious yawning, when someone yawns and you follow suit, seems to be linked to empathy—the ability to understand and feel affinity for another person's emotions. Several studies show that psychopaths, who by definition lack empathy, are immune to contagious yawning. It's also been suggested that this is a survival mechanism: when one person yawns, they suck the air out of the space they are in, so someone sharing that space automatically yawns to ensure they get their fair share of oxygen. While yawning may be one of science's great mysteries, if you're a contagious yawner, you can at least be fairly sure you're not a psychopath!

Why do we close our eyes to sleep?

Recent research has shown that the eye's role in synchronizing our circadian rhythm is more significant than previously thought, and this may help explain why we close our eyes during sleep.

Our eyes perform two essential tasks: as well as helping us navigate the world around us, they monitor and measure the light that controls our circadian rhythm (see pages 22–23). This rhythm is disrupted if the light we receive is too little, too much, or seen at the wrong time, leaving the internal clock "confused" about the time of day. By closing our eyes to sleep, we stop light from entering the eye and prompting the clock to wake us.

Closing our eyes to sleep also protects delicate eye structures. During the day, we blink to clear dust and debris and keep the surface of our eyes lubricated. When we sleep, our muscles relax and we don't blink, so closing our eyes overcomes any issues this might cause.

Some people are unable to shut their eyelids fully at night. This condition, known as nocturnal lagophthalmos, can be caused by skin disorders or problems with the eyelid structure but most often by conditions affecting facial nerves, such as Bell's palsy, where the facial muscles suffer temporary paralysis. If you have red, itchy, or painful eyes on waking, or if you have been told that your eyes don't close while you sleep, speak to your optician or doctor. Treatment options include eye drops or, in some cases, surgery may be necessary.

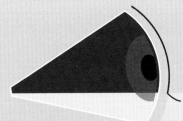

20% of people sleep with their eyes partially or fully open

Why do I grind my teeth when I sleep?

Do you wake up with a headache or tightness in the jaw or have very sensitive teeth? You might be suffering from sleep bruxism—the clenching or grinding of your teeth during the night.

Bruxism affects around 1 in 10 people, although many don't realize until their sleep partner comments or their dentist notices particular patterns of wear on their teeth. The muscles of the jaw are among the strongest in the body, and when you grind your teeth, these muscles go into hyperfunction and become constricted. This can lead to tension headaches, tooth fractures, changes to face shape, and jaw pain.

For about 70 percent of sufferers, bruxism stems from stress and anxiety, as teeth clenching and holding tension in the jaw and neck are common stress responses. For the other 30 percent, it appears to be genetic, comes down to bone structure, or occurs alongside another sleep disorder.

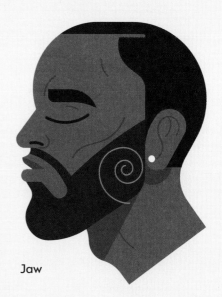

Jaw

Tension-beating massage
Take the index and middle fingers of both hands. Using fingertips, gently massage the muscles of the jaw, the temples, and the neck on both sides of your face in a circular motion. Whenever you feel tension and pain, massage each location for up to a minute at a time.

HOW TO MANAGE BRUXISM

• **A dentist** specially trained in dental sleep medicine can issue you a mouth guard to decompress the jaw. This will help reduce tension and pain as you sleep.

• **If you suspect stress**, and/or anxiety may be to blame, look at ways to relax or seek support—a course of CBTI (see pages 130–131) may help you manage your responses to stress.

• **If you suffer** from another sleep disorder, such as obstructive sleep apnea (see page 75), addressing the underlying causes of this could also relieve your bruxism.

• **For severe cases**, botox injections, which relax the jaw muscles involved in teeth grinding, could help.

• **Self-massage** can relieve constriction of the muscles in the jaw, temples, and neck—see below.

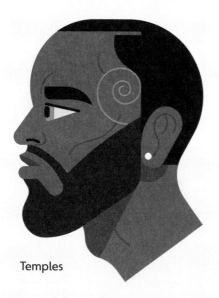

Temples

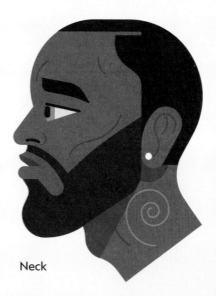

Neck

Why does my body stay asleep and immobile after my mind has woken up?

The experience of feeling awake but unable to move can be genuinely frightening, but what causes it?
The state known as sleep paralysis is fairly common and has been linked to conditions such as narcolepsy, PTSD, panic attacks, and seizure disorders. Other triggers may be lack of sleep, sleep disturbances, jet lag, or shift work.

During a normal night's sleep, as you enter REM sleep, the brain tells the nervous system that it's time to relax the muscles. This is because REM is a highly active brain state where dreaming takes place, so you become temporarily paralyzed to prevent your body from acting out dreams. Similar to experiencing the sensation of falling in your sleep (see page 72), sleep paralysis happens when the switch between REM and waking is delayed—meaning your body is still "paralyzed" but your brain has become conscious. This can often feel worse if it happens during a particularly vivid dream, because your brain is briefly unsure about what is and isn't real.

Although it's unsettling, you are not in any danger, and the experience may only last for seconds. (The average duration of an episode is around six minutes.) Nearly 8 percent of people will have at least one episode of sleep

Sleep paralysis process
During sleep paralysis, the brain wakes from REM sleep, but there is a delay in the "wake-up" message reaching the body's sleep centers, so they think you are still asleep and keep your limbs immobilized.

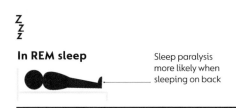

In REM sleep

Sleep paralysis more likely when sleeping on back

paralysis during their lifetime, although it is significantly more prevalent among young adults.

Another aspect of sleep paralysis is the "incubus phenomenon"—a feeling of pressure on your chest, sometimes accompanied by breathing difficulties, which probably results from a reduction in muscle activity. In folklore, an incubus was a male demon who sought out sleeping females to seduce, lying on top of them to immobilize them. This type of supernatural legend occurs in many cultural traditions and was most likely created to explain what we know today to be a simple physiological response.

WHAT SHOULD I DO?

The priority is to prevent a sleep paralysis episode becoming a source of anxiety that could affect your sleep longer term. Episodes can be distressing, but they do pass. As stress is a key trigger, relaxation before bedtime is vital. Also, maintaining good sleep hygiene has been shown to decrease the frequency of episodes—see pages 34–35.

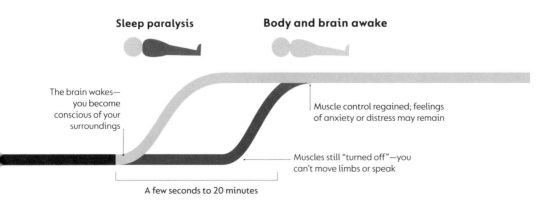

Sleep paralysis

Body and brain awake

The brain wakes—you become conscious of your surroundings

Muscle control regained; feelings of anxiety or distress may remain

Muscles still "turned off"—you can't move limbs or speak

A few seconds to 20 minutes

What causes the feeling of falling when I'm going to sleep?

You're just drifting off to sleep when suddenly you feel as if you are falling, and your body automatically jolts. This is known as a hypnic jerk, and there are several theories as to what causes it.

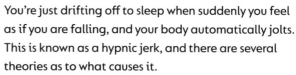

Hypnic jerks are a type of natural involuntary muscle movement in the legs called myoclonus—the same reflex that causes hiccups. The majority of us have them at some time or another, although people experience them differently: some feel like they are falling off the top of a building or out of bed, while others undergo an accompanying visual hallucination or an all-over body twitch.

One theory about the cause of these jerks is that when we are falling asleep, there are two systems in the brain in play—one is alert and the other acts as a sleep switch. Hypnic jerks occur when the body gets caught transitioning between the two, almost like a neurological battle between consciousness and unconsciousness.

SURVIVAL MECHANISM

Another hypothesis is that hypnic jerks are a hardwired survival mechanism that helped our primate ancestors ensure they were secured safely in their trees before relaxing and falling deeply asleep or that woke them up to check for nearby predators.

Of course, because hypnic jerks occur randomly as the body falls asleep, it could just be down to something as simple as the body preparing itself for rest—a physical consequence of our muscles relaxing.

If hypnic jerks stop you from getting to sleep, speak to your doctor to rule out restless legs syndrome (see page 95) or sleep-related leg cramps; both are treatable.

Hypnic jerks
occur in

70%

of people, and
10% of us may
experience
them daily

" " _____

Although the sensation of
falling can feel alarming,
it's simply an involuntary
reflex and doesn't cause
you any harm.

Why do I snore?

Have you ever been startled awake by the sound of a pneumatic drill, only to realize the noise was coming from you? Snoring can interrupt our sleep and that of those around us, but why does it happen?

When we sleep, the muscles in our throat and mouth relax. In snorers, these relaxed tissues sag into the windpipe, partially blocking it. As we breathe in and out, air is forced over and around these tissues, making them flap and vibrate—often noisily.

Snoring affects around 51 percent of men and 40 percent of women, and you are more likely to snore if you are overweight, smoke, drink alcohol, take sleep medication, or sleep on your back—all of which can overrelax the throat muscles during sleep. Those with allergies or frequent sinus infections may also be more prone to snoring, as a blocked nose further restricts airflow.

Although disruptive, snoring in itself isn't dangerous unless it's a symptom of obstructive sleep apnea (OSA, see opposite page), a potentially serious condition that requires medical treatment.

SNORING QUICK FIXES

• Sleep on your side to keep airways more open—a pregnancy pillow may help you stay in position.

• A wedge pillow under the neck raises the head and prevents throat muscles from sagging too much.

• A nasal spray can reduce any congestion in your nose and sinuses.

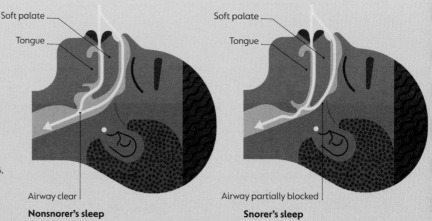

The mechanics of snoring

If the airway is fully open during sleep, breathing is normal and snoring does not occur. The main tissues that disturb airflow and cause snoring are the nasal passageways, the soft palate, and the tongue.

Soft palate

Tongue

Airway clear

Nonsnorer's sleep

Soft palate

Tongue

Airway partially blocked

Snorer's sleep

Why does my partner seem to gasp for air in his sleep?

A pattern of snoring punctuated by gasping or spluttering could be obstructive sleep apnea (OSA), a potentially serious condition.

OSA occurs when throat muscles sag so much during sleep that the airway becomes blocked, waking the sufferer briefly in order to take a breath. This repeated pattern causes chronic fatigue—and long term, can lead to serious illnesses such as type 2 diabetes, high blood pressure, heart attack, and mental illness.

Anyone can suffer OSA, but a major risk factor is being overweight, as fatty tissues in the throat and mouth are likely to block more of the airway when they sag.

DIAGNOSING AND TREATING OSA

OSA is diagnosed by a sleep study to measure incidents over a night. Depending on the cause, your doctor may recommend a CPAP (continuous positive airway pressure) device, a mask to keep the airway open; a jawline-altering mouth guard; or lifestyle changes such as losing weight, quitting smoking, or drinking less alcohol.

The OSA cycle

When a sufferer's airway becomes fully blocked by soft tissue, the body is starved of oxygen, and this emergency jolts the person awake to take a breath. This constant cycle of brief suffocations and traumatic awakenings puts all the body's systems under severe strain and causes damage to the memory-storing hippocampus region of the brain.

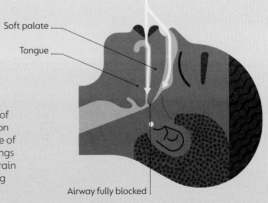

Soft palate

Tongue

Airway fully blocked

OSA sleep

Why does my temperature fluctuate when I sleep?

Feeling too hot—or too cold—is not conducive to sleep. How many of us have stuck our legs out of the covers to cool down, only to wake in the middle of the night with freezing toes?

As we sleep, our body temperature changes throughout the night, and there's an important reason for this. Body temperature is controlled by our circadian rhythm (see pages 22–23), with core temperature rising and falling by a few degrees over a 24-hour period. The brain uses these changes to help it regulate the sleep/wake cycle, signaling the body to release hormones that either wake us or send us to sleep.

The timing of these fluctuations is mainly governed by the changes in natural light over each 24-hour period. A few hours before waking up, your temperature rises slightly as dawn approaches. This triggers a release of the energizing hormone cortisol to help wake you up. Your temperature continues to rise, peaking around late

Highs and lows

Although the body's core temperature fluctuates by only a couple of degrees, these small changes are enough to set off the hormonal signals that control our cycle of waking and sleeping.

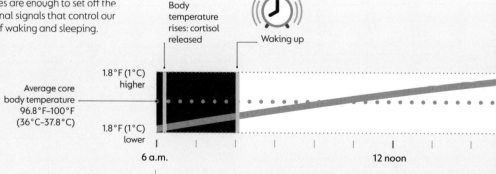

Body temperature rises: cortisol released

Waking up

1.8°F (1°C) higher

Average core body temperature 96.8°F–100°F (36°C–37.8°C)

1.8°F (1°C) lower

6 a.m.

12 noon

afternoon, before dropping again when the light fades. This generates the release of the hormone melatonin, which winds down alertness and prepares you for sleep. Body temperature continues to drop and is at its lowest a few hours after you fall asleep—which accounts for those freezing toes at 2 a.m.!

Core body temperature can also fluctuate in response to the activities you engage in, illnesses, the temperature of the environment around you, and—for those who menstruate—their monthly cycle. If you are too hot before bed, it will be harder to fall asleep, as your body won't release enough melatonin. If you are too cold in the early morning, your body won't release enough cortisol—which may explain why we struggle more to get up on cold winter mornings.

For better-quality sleep, start by getting your room temperature right (see page 181), and be aware of the impact of your bedtime routine on core temperature—a hot bath or very strenuous exercise could interfere with melatonin production and make it harder to drop off.

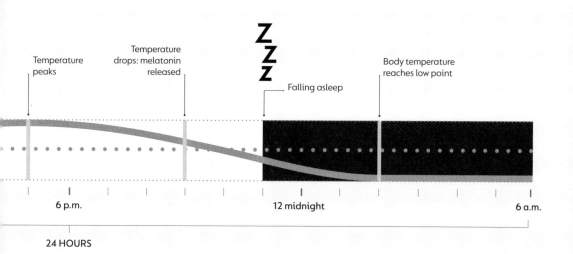

Temperature peaks

Temperature drops: melatonin released

Z Z Z

Falling asleep

Body temperature reaches low point

6 p.m.

12 midnight

6 a.m.

24 HOURS

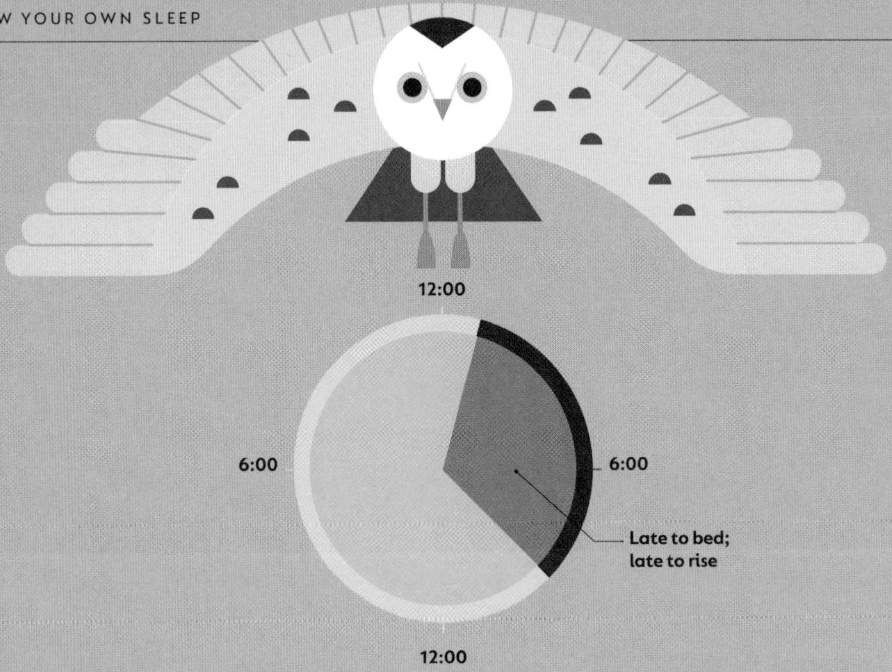

12:00

6:00

6:00

Late to bed;
late to rise

12:00

Why am I more nocturnal than others I know?

If you're still wide awake and full of energy when everyone in the house is sound asleep, it's likely that biologically you are a "night owl."
Sleep, like other body functions, is governed by our circadian rhythms, and the exact timings of an individual's sleep/wake cycle vary from person to person. This variation is known as your "chronotype," and it influences not only the timing of your sleep, but other daily activities, such as eating and exercise.

There are two main chronotypes: "early birds" and "night owls." Early birds are early risers, functioning better in the mornings but ready for sleep relatively early; night owls rise later and take longer to reach peak functioning, but then remain alert until later into the night. Although there are extremes at either end of the scale, most people fall somewhere in between the two and are known as "intermediates."

GETTING THE MOST OUT OF YOUR CHRONOTYPE

A chronotype is genetically programmed—you can't reset it. However, by understanding your chronotype, you can ensure you embrace rather than fight it. For instance, early birds may schedule important meetings for the morning and leave routine tasks for later in the day, when they are running out of mental steam. Happily, there is a growing trend for employers to recognize that not everybody performs best on a 9-to-5 schedule. Night owls benefit especially from more flexible working hours: one study found that allowing them to start work just half an hour later resulted in a significant drop in sick leave.

OWL OR BIRD?

Familiarity with your own sleep habits can help you adjust your lifestyle to better suit your chronotype. Try keeping a sleep journal (see pages 36–37) and pay attention to the following indicators:

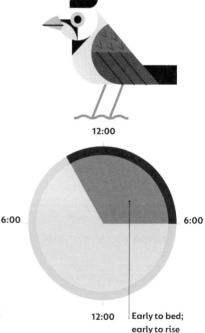

12:00

6:00   6:00

12:00   Early to bed;
            early to rise

• **Alertness on waking** A good gauge of chronotype is how quickly your brain wakes up. If you repeatedly hit "snooze" or sleep through the alarm, you are likely more of a night owl.

• **Focus and concentration** Early birds peak early in the day, then concentration tails off gradually. Night owls start later but can retain their focus late into the evening and night.

• **Physical performance** Early birds peak physically in the morning; performing physical tasks or doing exercise at the optimum time for you will help you avoid injury and strains.

• **Sleep time** If they go to bed earlier than usual, early birds tend to fall asleep easily. For night owls, early nights are futile; it's almost impossible for them to fall asleep before midnight.

Yoga routine for sleep

Ten minutes before bed, take a yoga mat and find a quiet space. Begin by lying on your back and breathe in through your nose for a count of three until your abdomen feels full, hold for a count of two, then exhale gently through your mouth for a count of three. Continue breathing slowly and deeply as you work through the routine.

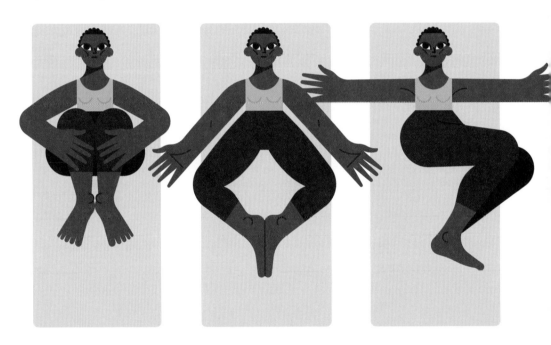

KNEES TO CHEST
Gently draw your knees in toward your chest and clasp your hands around them while you focus on your breathing. Hold this pose for up to one minute before releasing your knees, keeping them bent, and placing the soles of your feet on the mat.

RECLINED BUTTERFLY POSE
Bring your arms down by your sides, palms facing up. Place the soles of your feet together and let your legs fall open. Focus on your breathing and hold this pose for up to one minute. Finish by bringing your legs back together, with the soles of your feet on the mat.

SUPINE TWIST
Stretch your arms out in a "T" shape. Send your knees to one side and turn your head to look in the opposite direction. Slowly bring your knees back to center. Repeat for the other side. Continue for up to one minute, then bring your knees to center to finish.

Can yoga help with sleep?

Yoga is a philosophy and form of exercise that combines physical poses with controlled breathing. Some types of yoga are physically demanding and energizing, while others are relaxing and meditative, making them great for aiding sleep.

All yoga disciplines involve a form of deep, conscious breathing called pranayama. Pranayama not only helps slow the heart rate, but also stimulates the vagus, the largest nerve in the body, which runs from the brain to the stomach. This nerve plays a key role in activating the parasympathetic nervous system, which is responsible for calming our stress response. Pranayama has been shown to reduce tension and hyperalertness and promote relaxation.

SLOWING THE MIND

Some forms of yoga also help you reach the ideal brain states required for sleep. Hatha yoga is slow-paced, restorative, and relaxing; nidrā yoga involves guided meditation to help you enter a hypnotic state. One study has shown that nidrā yoga can increase a person's ability to enter the deepest, delta-wave state of sleep.

Yoga is widely accessible; you can choose to learn at a class or via various online or digital platforms. Although nidrā yoga is always a guided practice, the simple pranayama exercise and hatha yoga poses on this page can be followed easily at home. Practice them last thing at night to complete your wind-down routine before sleep.

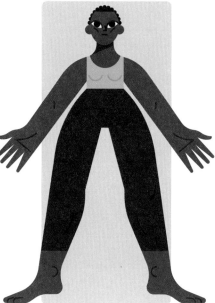

CORPSE POSE

Take your arms down to your sides, palms facing up. Relax your legs so they lie flat and slightly apart. Lie still and breathe deeply and gently for around one minute. You can either end here or, if you wish, repeat the routine of poses several more times.

When should I exercise for optimum sleep?

Exercise is essential for health and well-being, but the timing and intensity of exercise can impact sleep. Working in harmony with your body clock means you can get the most out of exercise and ensure good sleep. In general, exercise will increase sleep pressure (see page 108), helping you not only fall asleep, but stay asleep for longer.

- **Early morning** Cortisol levels in the body are naturally high. Cortisol helps lower inflammation, improving the body's rest and repair functions, so this can make recovery from an early-morning workout easier.

- **Afternoon/early evening** Exercising between 3 p.m. and 7 p.m. is not only good for sleep, but can maximize the physical benefits of your workout, because coordination and muscle strength usually peak during

Sync with your rhythms

Taking into account your circadian rhythms when you plan exercise means you can maximize the benefits of being active while still ensuring great sleep.

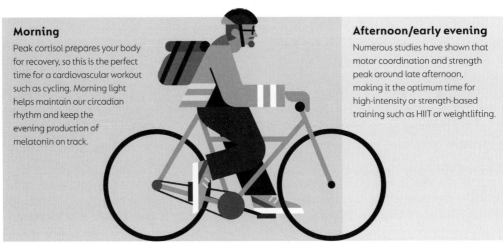

Morning

Peak cortisol prepares your body for recovery, so this is the perfect time for a cardiovascular workout such as cycling. Morning light helps maintain our circadian rhythm and keep the evening production of melatonin on track.

Afternoon/early evening

Numerous studies have shown that motor coordination and strength peak around late afternoon, making it the optimum time for high-intensity or strength-based training such as HIIT or weightlifting.

this time frame. Bear in mind, however, that the optimum time for exercise can also depend on your chronotype (see pages 78–79), so an hour on either side of this window may work better for you.

• **Late evening/night** Late-night workouts can significantly interfere with sleep, so winding down before bed is key. Physical exertion releases adrenaline and cortisol, which raises body temperature and keeps you in a state of alertness. These hormones also delay the release of melatonin, preventing you from feeling sleepy. If your schedule means that this is the only time you can exercise, try to leave a couple of hours between finishing a workout and going to bed to allow your mind and body to wind down. A cool shower will also reduce your temperature, preparing your body for sleep onset.

REST AND REPAIR

Human growth hormone is necessary for muscle repair, and during deep sleep, levels reach their peak in your body. Interruptions to the deeper stages of sleep can mean the body misses out on vital opportunities for repair, which is especially important after exercise. Sufficient, good-quality sleep will ensure that you maintain good muscle health and lower your risk of injury when you exercise.

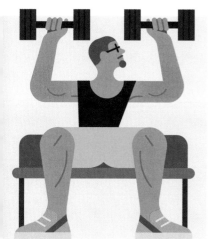

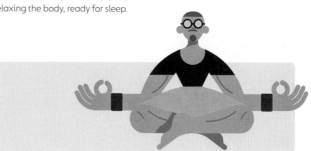

Late evening

Ideally, avoid exercise that's too strenuous as bedtime approaches. Gentle, mindful exercise such as hatha yoga can help you focus on relaxing the body, ready for sleep.

Can a lack of sleep affect my immune system?

The immune system function is boosted by sleep, so it's important—now more than ever—to get enough quality sleep to be able to ward off illness and disease.

During sleep, our immune system is highly active, releasing cytokines—proteins that the body needs to fight infections and inflammation. Being deprived of sleep means that reduced production of cytokines lowers resistance to bacteria and increases the risk of illness.

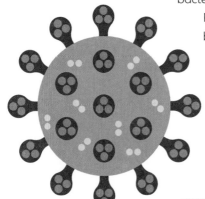

Poor sleep can also be a problem when it comes to beating viruses. When the immune system identifies a virally infected cell, it activates T-cells to attach to and destroy the cell. When scientists compared T-cells from healthy volunteers who slept all night to those in volunteers who stayed awake, they found that the sleepers' T-cells showed higher levels of activation than those of the sleep-deprived.

THE ROLE OF CHRONIC STRESS

When the body is put under stress, it releases cortisol. Although cortisol usually helps fight inflammation, chronic stress means that the body is subjected to consistently high cortisol levels, which dials down the immune system response. This is because, over time, the body becomes resistant to cortisol, and the hormone no longer fights inflammation, but actually triggers it. We know that chronic stress interferes with sleep in other ways, too (see pages 208–209), so finding effective ways to manage and reduce it is key to the good sleep that leads to a healthy immune system. For effective relaxation techniques, see pages 80–81 and 124–125.

Is my thyroid to blame for my poor sleep?

The thyroid gland secretes hormones that help regulate many body processes, and when it isn't working properly, this can impair our health—and our sleep.

The thyroid produces the hormones triiodothyronine (T3) and thyroxine (T4), which are involved in controlling the metabolism and the regulation of body temperature and heart rate. Hypothyroidism occurs when the thyroid doesn't produce enough T3 and T4. It's relatively common, especially in older women, and often causes weight gain, which can in turn lead to snoring and sleep apnea. This condition is treated with hormone-replacing medication, and once T3 and T4 levels normalize, many symptoms disappear or become easier to manage.

With hyperthyroidism, the thyroid produces too much hormone. It's also more common in women, but it usually occurs at a younger age. The excess hormone overstimulates the nervous system, leading to anxiety and increased heart rate, which can make it harder to fall asleep and may also cause night sweats. There are a range of treatments, and once under control, some of the symptoms linked to poor sleep may disappear. However, if insomnia has taken hold, it may need to be tackled separately, for instance, with a course of CBTI (see pages 132–133).

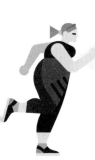
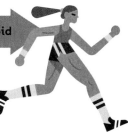

Underactive thyroid

- Tiredness
- Feeling cold
- Weight gain
- Poor concentration
- Depression

Overactive thyroid

- Anxiety
- Increased heart rate
- Insomnia
- Night sweats

Will lack of sleep affect my weight?

When sleep deprived, we feel low in energy, and it's tempting to rely on high-energy, sugary snacks to keep us going. But lack of sleep affects our food choices in other, more profound ways.

A higher BMI (body mass index—a measure of whether a person's weight is healthy) has been shown to be associated with poor sleep, so could it be that it's actually sleep deprivation that's somehow making us fat? The answer is a resounding "yes." In a study, just one night

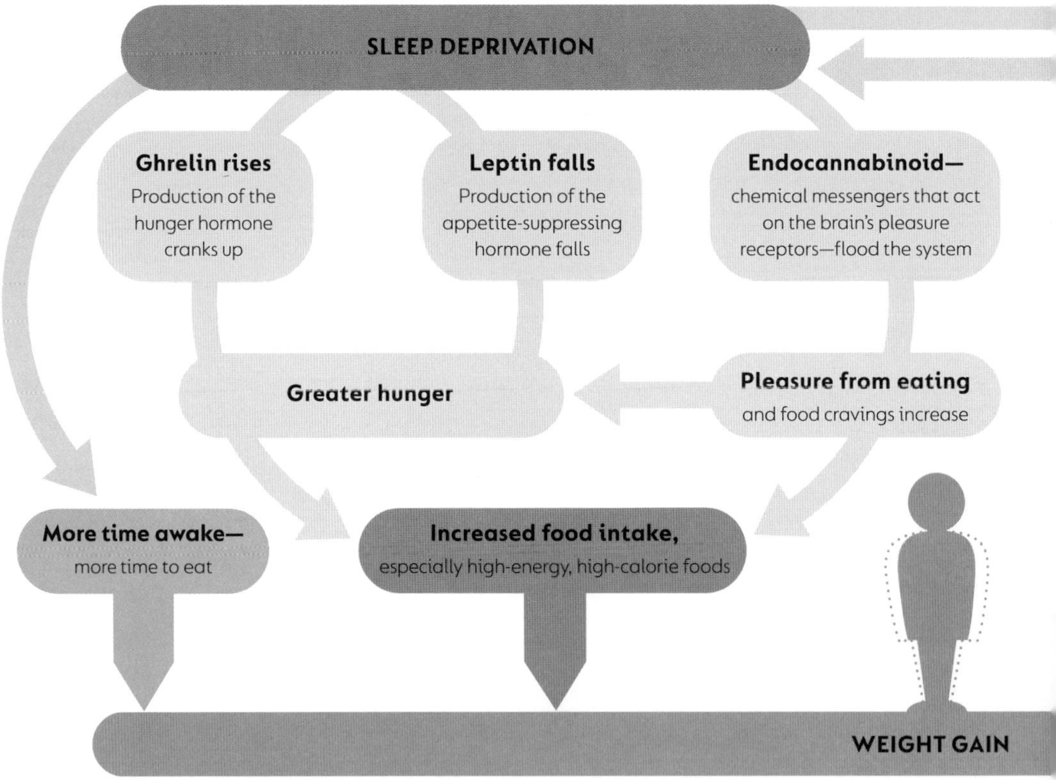

SLEEP DEPRIVATION

Ghrelin rises
Production of the hunger hormone cranks up

Leptin falls
Production of the appetite-suppressing hormone falls

Endocannabinoid—
chemical messengers that act on the brain's pleasure receptors—flood the system

Greater hunger

Pleasure from eating
and food cravings increase

More time awake—
more time to eat

Increased food intake,
especially high-energy, high-calorie foods

WEIGHT GAIN

of poor sleep (defined as less than five hours) led to people eating up to 385 extra calories the next day. Those calories quickly add up, and a month of poor sleep can lead to an increase in body fat of around 2 pounds (1 kg).

HOW SLEEP AFFECTS EATING

When we are fully rested, leptin (the appetite-suppressing hormone) is high, and ghrelin (the hormone responsible for hunger) is low. Lack of sleep reverses this, so you are hungrier than usual when you wake. Poor sleep also raises the level of endocannabinoids in the blood. These brain chemicals magnify ghrelin-induced cravings, making it difficult to resist instantly satisfying junk food. This is why when you're sleep deprived and have a choice between a spinach omelet or a chocolate donut, you feel powerfully driven toward the latter.

Less sleep also means more time awake, and with our brain's reward centers in overdrive, we become highly susceptible to any food cues, eating far more than we would normally. Added to this is the fatigue we feel after a bad night's sleep, which saps our motivation to exercise. Moving less means burning fewer calories, so all the extra food is stored as fat. Gaining weight can turn a relatively mild sleeping issue into a more serious condition, such as sleep apnea (see page 75).

BETTER SLEEP FOR WEIGHT MANAGEMENT

Increasing the amount of sleep you get will quickly restore leptin and ghrelin levels to normal and prevent your brain from turning itself into a calorie-seeking missile. More sleep also means more energy and, often, a lighter mood—helping you find the drive needed to address your diet and exercise positively in the longer term.

Poor sleep, poor eating

Recent research indicates that insufficient sleep plays havoc with important appetite-controlling hormones in the body. In combination with the other consequences of poor sleep, it's a recipe for weight gain.

Chronic tiredness
leads to low energy and low mood

Body not tired—
sleepiness delayed

Inactivity
No desire to exercise

Will an orgasm help me sleep better?

For the majority of people, having an orgasm appears to bring on sleepiness, but is there any science to explain this effect?

The combination of hormones that are released when you experience orgasm all play a role in relaxing your mind and body, as well as contributing to the biological processes needed for sleep—making it more likely you'll fall into a restful slumber.

Oxytocin, known as the "love hormone," promotes feelings of affection and also counters the effects of cortisol in the body, soothing and de-stressing us and allowing sleep to come more easily.

Serotonin, the "happy hormone," not only encourages a good mood and relaxation postorgasm, but is also required by the body in order to make melatonin, the hormone that signals to the body that we are sleepy.

Prolactin serves many functions, one of which is to encourage sleep onset. It may cause sleepiness after sex—research has shown that men release up to four times more prolactin than women when they orgasm.

But it's not only our hormones that signal it's time for sleep. During orgasm, the parts of our brain that are involved in logical thinking also switch off—priming the mind to be free from worries and decision-making and instead to zone out and get ready for rest.

If you struggle with getting to sleep, having an orgasm at night, when your body is already in sleep-preparation mode, could very well be an effective way to drift off into a relaxed and satisfying sleep.

BETTER WITH TWO?

All orgasms promote sleep to some degree, but studies have shown that those achieved during sex with a partner appear to have a greater sleep-inducing effect—particularly in males—compared to those experienced through solo sexual activity.

" " _____

The hormones released
during orgasm not only
help us sleep, they also
naturally relieve pain
and reduce stress.

Why is my sleep so affected by my monthly cycle?

You may find that you experience poor sleep before and during your period, as well as around ovulation—this is brought on by hormonal changes in the body.

Just before and after a period begins, progesterone and estrogen levels are at their lowest, inhibiting the release of melatonin, the sleepiness hormone. This can result in problems with both falling and staying asleep. This usually passes by around day seven as hormone levels rise but can recur during ovulation (approximately day 14 of a 28-day cycle) when estrogen peaks—it stimulates the nervous system and increases wakefulness. Sleep improves toward day 21, only to be disrupted again as you reach day 28, and hormones dip again.

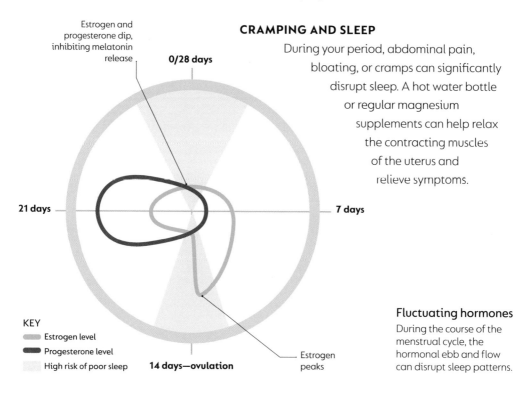

Estrogen and progesterone dip, inhibiting melatonin release

0/28 days

21 days

7 days

14 days—ovulation

Estrogen peaks

KEY
- Estrogen level
- Progesterone level
- High risk of poor sleep

CRAMPING AND SLEEP

During your period, abdominal pain, bloating, or cramps can significantly disrupt sleep. A hot water bottle or regular magnesium supplements can help relax the contracting muscles of the uterus and relieve symptoms.

Fluctuating hormones
During the course of the menstrual cycle, the hormonal ebb and flow can disrupt sleep patterns.

Will a lack of sleep affect my libido and fertility?

The hormone testosterone plays a key role in sex drive and sperm production. Poor sleep inhibits testosterone levels, and too much or too little of this hormone can disrupt sleep.

Testosterone is the sex hormone mainly responsible for many of the typical physical characteristics of males. Too little testosterone in the body can lead to problems such as erectile dysfunction, poor mood, weight gain, and reduced sperm count.

Testosterone levels rise as you fall asleep, reaching their peak during the first bout of REM sleep. Poor sleep, and the consequent lack of REM, can therefore lead to a reduction in testosterone production.

Low testosterone—which can be the result of injury, illness, or old age—also seems to play a role in poor sleep for some men. One study of men aged 65 and over showed that those with low testosterone spent less time in slow-wave sleep and had more episodes of nighttime waking. Low testosterone can also lead to weight gain, increasing the risk of developing sleep-disrupting snoring or sleep apnea.

Too much testosterone can also interfere with sleep—the use of steroids that contain the hormone has been associated with insomnia.

Although the complex relationship between sleep and testosterone is not yet fully understood, it's clear that good sleep is important to maintain the healthy testosterone levels that are key to male sexual well-being.

One study showed men who had four hours' sleep had

10–15%

less testosterone than men who slept for eight hours

How can I manage my chronic pain to sleep better?

Up to **88 percent of chronic pain sufferers report that they also struggle with poor-quality sleep, which in turn can ramp up their symptoms and worsen pain.**

A range of medical issues can cause chronic pain. Fibromyalgia, multiple sclerosis, rheumatoid arthritis, osteoarthritis, nerve damage, and cancer are all leading causes of persistent pain, although sometimes it occurs with no identifiable cause. The relationship between pain and sleep is a two-way street: pain leads to poor sleep, and poor sleep increases our perception of pain. A lack of deep sleep also disrupts the body's ability to fight pain. It inhibits the production of the hormones prolactin and HGH, which have anti-inflammatory properties and are

Sleep loss/pain cycle

Poor sleep not only increases our vulnerability to and perception of pain, but pain itself can be the trigger for problems falling and staying asleep—perpetuating the negative relationship between sleep and pain.

PAIN

Trouble falling asleep

In bed with no distractions, the perception of pain can increase. The more you feel pain, the more difficult it is to fall asleep.

Trouble staying asleep

Pain triggers a stress response in the body, heightening our arousal and increasing the likelihood we will wake.

LACK OF SLEEP

Poor sleep increases pain sensitivity and reduces the body's ability to manage pain.

vital to the body's repair processes—and this further adds to the burden of chronic pain.

The automatic response we have to pain is to tense our muscles. For chronic-pain sufferers, muscle tension can therefore seem normal and may not even be something they are aware of. However, this tension can make the experience of pain worse, so learning to relax can be an effective way to reduce symptoms.

RELAX TO BREAK THE CYCLE

Progressive muscle relaxation is a practice whereby you relax the muscles of the body in turn, which is proven to help with pain management. Studies have shown that it can decrease the sensation of pain and improve sleep. To see if it works for you, you'll need around 10 minutes for the following exercise:

1. Lie on your back in bed, or on a yoga mat, and take a minute to allow your breathing to come to a slow, steady rhythm. Be aware of your inhales and exhales.

2. Beginning with your left foot, tense the muscles in your foot tightly, inhaling slowly, and hold for a count of five. Exhale and release all the tension in the foot—your muscles will feel a sudden relaxing sensation. Repeat this process twice more before repeating for the right foot.

3. Repeat this gentle process of breathing, tensing, then releasing the muscles all the way up your body in the following sequence: calves, thighs, buttocks, stomach, hands, arms, chest, shoulders, neck, and face.

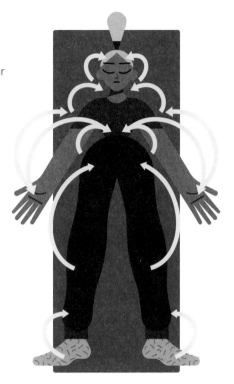

Gradual relaxation

The progressive muscle relaxation exercise (see left) works by focusing on one area of the body at a time. Starting from your feet, tense and release the muscles first on the left side, then on the right, before moving on to the next group of muscles. Gradually work up to your head, as shown above.

Why do I move around so much while I'm asleep?

Waking after a night of tossing and turning can leave you feeling as if you've hardly slept at all.

First, it's normal and beneficial to shift position during the night: this maintains blood circulation and prevents numbness or pins and needles. We move around during all sleep stages except the REM stage, when the muscles are temporarily paralyzed. During the lighter sleep of Stages 1 and 2, your movements merely cause "mini arousals," which don't wake you fully, so you immediately fall back asleep.

PROBLEMATIC MOVEMENT

If you do recall tossing and turning and don't feel rested when you wake, it's most likely that you were roused from Stage 3, the deepest level of sleep. A variety of factors could be responsible, including strenuous exercise close to bedtime, anxiety, or being too hot. Medical conditions such as sleep apnea, restless legs syndrome, or chronic pain can also trigger nighttime agitation.

Another cause could be a condition called periodic limb movement disorder (PLMD). This causes prolonged periods of arm and leg twitching, lasting 20–40 seconds at a time—disturbing you and putting your sleep partner at risk of an unexpected whack! Unlike restless legs syndrome, PLMD only occurs during sleep. Scientists have identified that people carrying a specific gene are at higher risk of PLMD, although high blood pressure, overstimulation, and anxiety also seem to be linked.

If you suspect you have this condition, see your doctor. Reducing stress is key to lowering your arousal level and stabilizing blood pressure. Caffeine also worsens PLMD symptoms, so avoid all caffeinated food and drink for the four to five hours before bed.

The average healthy adult sleeper moves their body around

50–60

times a night

Why are my legs painful and restless at night?

If you get the irresistible urge to move your legs in bed at night, you're not alone. Restless legs syndrome (RLS)—a neurological disorder that disrupts sleep—is a surprisingly common condition.

RLS occurs most often when the body is inactive, which is why it is usually experienced in bed at night. Some experts believe that RLS is due to a problem in the part of the brain that controls movement and muscle activity, but studies have not yet proved this conclusively. Recent clinical research suggests that low iron levels in the brain may be responsible. However, as yet there is no easy way to test brain iron levels, so researchers are still some way off seeing the complete picture.

RLS can occur at any age and has a 60 percent chance of being inherited. Mostly, there's no obvious trigger, though for some, vitamin D deficiency, nerve damage, or sleep apnea may be linked to its onset. One in five women suffer RLS in pregnancy, possibly due to low iron and folate, and the condition usually fades after childbirth.

MANAGING RLS

A cure for RLS is still a work in progress, but there are some things you can try to alleviate symptoms:

• **A pillow** between your legs while you sleep may prevent nerve compression and make the legs more comfortable.

• **A walk** before bed, or stretching the leg muscles when symptoms are at their worst, can soothe symptoms.

• **Taking iron**, folate, or vitamin D can help some sufferers, but always consult your doctor before taking supplements.

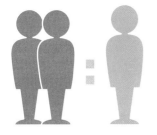

2 : 1

Women are twice as likely as men to experience RLS

What's the best position for me to sleep in?

We fall asleep in the position that feels best to us, then reposition ourselves in the night to maintain comfort, and some positions are better for us than others. Starting your night's sleep in a position that works for your specific needs could help you fall into a comfortable slumber and make a good night's rest more likely.

ON YOUR BACK

As long as your head, neck, and knees are well supported, sleeping on your back reduces strain on these areas, which is good for those who suffer joint stiffness. Placing a small pillow under your knees will support the natural curve of your lower spine and lessen back strain. Elevating your head slightly can also reduce the symptoms of acid reflux, and some even swear it wards off wrinkles (see pages 98–99). However, for snorers and those with sleep apnea, sleeping on your back will worsen these conditions.

ON YOUR FRONT

Sleeping on your front can stop you from snoring, but it causes your head to twist to one side for long periods, which places the most pressure on your neck and spine and can lead to trapped nerves. It may also cause lower back pain due to the relatively heavy middle part of your body pulling the spine downward out of its natural shape. It's better not to sleep on your front, but if you do, try putting a firm pillow under your stomach to support your spine.

ON YOUR SIDE

Sleeping on one side is best for most sleepers; it puts the least pressure on the spine and other joints and is best for snorers. However, the left and right sides are not created equal—studies show that left-side sleeping is best because

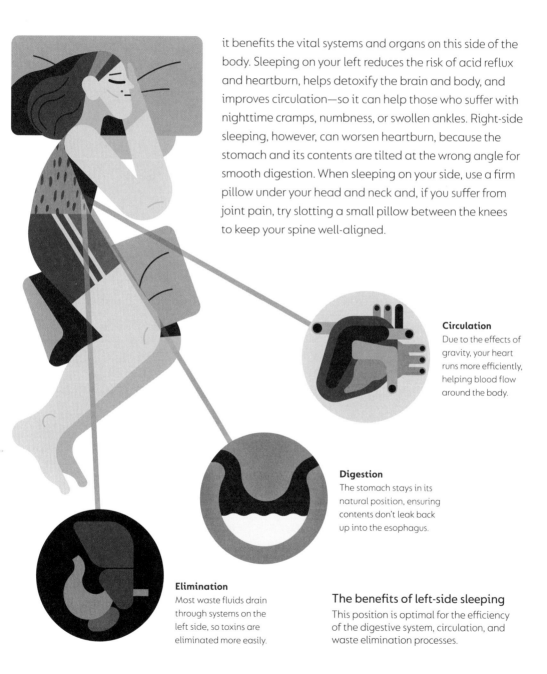

it benefits the vital systems and organs on this side of the body. Sleeping on your left reduces the risk of acid reflux and heartburn, helps detoxify the brain and body, and improves circulation—so it can help those who suffer with nighttime cramps, numbness, or swollen ankles. Right-side sleeping, however, can worsen heartburn, because the stomach and its contents are tilted at the wrong angle for smooth digestion. When sleeping on your side, use a firm pillow under your head and neck and, if you suffer from joint pain, try slotting a small pillow between the knees to keep your spine well-aligned.

Circulation
Due to the effects of gravity, your heart runs more efficiently, helping blood flow around the body.

Digestion
The stomach stays in its natural position, ensuring contents don't leak back up into the esophagus.

Elimination
Most waste fluids drain through systems on the left side, so toxins are eliminated more easily.

The benefits of left-side sleeping
This position is optimal for the efficiency of the digestive system, circulation, and waste elimination processes.

Is beauty sleep real?

You might think "beauty sleep" is a myth, but one look at the dark circles under your eyes after a poor night's sleep is enough to tell you that how we sleep can have a real effect on how we look.

There's genuine science behind the maxim that a full night of good-quality sleep will enhance our looks. Over the course of the night, the body performs important repair and regeneration functions. The later phase of sleep is when the majority of this rejuvenation takes place, so when you miss all or part of this phase, there are negative consequences. Also, disrupted sleep induces a stress response in the body, prompting the release of hormones that both interfere with the damage-repairing processes and trigger inflammation, which can affect skin by breaking down the proteins that keep it looking and feeling radiant and smooth.

Biological beauty treatment

This timeline shows that the longer you sleep, the more your body's self-repair system can take effect, especially as most of this vital process takes place in the third phase of sleep.

DURING SLEEP

 Skin damage repaired

During deep sleep, the hypothalamus releases growth hormone, which increases collagen production. Collagen keeps skin plump and prevents wrinkles from forming. A delay in falling asleep reduces growth hormone production.

 Antioxidants released

Melatonin levels increase between 2 a.m. and 4 a.m. As well as keeping you asleep, melatonin acts as an antioxidant to protect the skin from free radicals—unstable atoms that can attach to skin cells, causing inflammation and damage.

Poor sleep also causes blood to flow less efficiently around the body. This means that the blood lacks oxygen—which is what makes your complexion pasty, gray, and dull when you wake too early. Poor blood flow can also cause blood to pool in the area under the eyes, and because the skin here is so thin, the blood shows through as dark circles and puffiness. Getting enough sleep regularly is the most potent weapon in the long-term fight against premature skin aging, but to reduce eye bags and puffiness in the short term, try sleeping on your back with your head raised on an extra pillow—this allows gravity to drain the blood away instead of it getting stuck around the eye sockets.

IT'S IN THE GENES

Genes play a key role in the skin's appearance. People with skin that's inherently thinner or lighter-colored will have more visible dark circles when blood pools under their eyes. And no matter how assiduously we care for our skin, the aging process is inevitable and natural—production of skin-plumping collagen slows as we get older, and the outermost layer of skin becomes thinner.

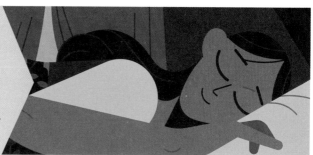

IN THE MORNING

Fully rested

After a full night's sleep, stress hormones are at their lowest, allowing anti-inflammatory melatonin and growth hormone to renew, repair, and detoxify skin cells.

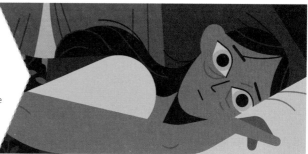

Insufficient sleep

Too little sleep reduces time spent in deep sleep, impacting growth hormone production. It also causes a spike in stress hormones adrenaline and cortisol, both of which interfere with cellular repair.

Can sleeping pills cure my sleep problem?

If you're sleep-deprived and in desperate need of a good night's rest, sleeping pills are a tempting option—but there are drawbacks.

Sleep medications aim to help you fall asleep more quickly and stay asleep for longer. Over-the-counter remedies usually contain antihistamines or herbal extracts such as valerian or lemon balm, which act as relaxants on brain and body. Prescription sleep medications, whether they are antidepressants, Z-drugs, or benzodiazepines, are powerful drugs that significantly affect brain and body functions.

MANUFACTURED SLEEP

The issue with long-term use of sleep medications is that they can create more problems than they solve. Antihistamines may leave you drowsy the next day, and too-frequent use can cause forgetfulness and headaches. Prescription-drug-induced sleep is not the same as the natural kind, as these drugs reduce both REM and the deep, restorative phases of the sleep cycle. In addition, nearly all prescribed sleep medications carry a risk of dependence and withdrawal symptoms, so their use must be closely managed by a medical professional.

Sleep medications can be useful for short-term issues, such as when recovering from a medical procedure, but for most problems, there are better long-term strategies, such as CBTI, good sleep hygiene, or relaxation techniques. Always speak to your doctor before starting any course of sleep medication, even over-the-counter remedies.

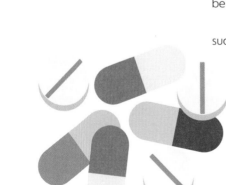

Can melatonin supplements help me sleep?

Melatonin, the sleepiness hormone, plays a key role in the sleep/wake cycle, so could taking it as a supplement be useful for those who struggle to fall and stay asleep?
Melatonin is naturally produced by the body in response to changes in daylight. Around two hours before bed— provided the light has dimmed—its release is triggered, helping us feel sleepy. There's evidence to suggest that melatonin supplements can provide relief for adult insomnia sufferers, helping them fall asleep faster. It also seems to relieve the disrupting effects of jet lag and shift work. Taking melatonin appears to be safe, with fewer side effects than many other sleep medications. It works best as a short-term aid; taking it over a longer period may interfere with your body's own natural melatonin production.

There is an ongoing debate about giving melatonin supplements to children. Because melatonin naturally drops with the onset of adolescence, there is some concern that long-term use in children may delay or disrupt puberty.

In many countries, melatonin is available over the counter, but the amount of hormone in each product can vary greatly. One study of melatonin supplements found that their actual melatonin content ranged from -83 percent to +478 percent of the labeled amount. If you are considering using supplements, it's safest to do so under the supervision of a doctor or sleep professional.

" "

Exposure to daylight is just as effective as melatonin supplements in triggering the body's natural sleepiness.

How does my mood affect my sleep?

A night of poor sleep is likely to affect your mood the next day—and your state of mind then has the potential to affect the sleep you get the following night.

Our thoughts, behaviors, and physical feelings are all intimately connected and feed into our state of mind. Negative emotions, such as fear and anger, can trigger the biological stress response and flood your body with adrenaline and cortisol, making it difficult for you to get to sleep and stay asleep and more likely that you will wake earlier the following morning in a low mood.

GOOD OR BAD MOOD?

Interestingly, it's also possible that you could experience a night of disrupted sleep, but if your mood is good, you may not perceive it as such. From the perspective of the nervous system, anxiety, fear, excitement, or joy are not that different—they are all heightened states of arousal. The difference is in how your brain interprets them. Anxiety is experienced as a negative emotion, so a physical manifestation of it, such as butterflies in the stomach, is interpreted as upsetting or uncomfortable. Excitement is a positive emotion, so those same stomach butterflies don't feel like a problem. So a sleepless night before an eagerly anticipated vacation is perceived completely differently to one before, say, a big test.

BOOSTING MOOD FOR BETTER SLEEP

Many things can affect mood through the day: natural peaks in energy levels; family or work pressures; and even how, when, and what we eat. One way to track whether your moods are affecting your sleep is to keep a daily mood journal. A key component of your sleep journal (see pages 36–37) should be recording your moods and any accompanying physical feelings or emotions. This will help you detect patterns that could be at the root of your poor sleep.

Research shows that those who experience more positive emotions also report better sleep quality—so finding strategies to help you manage negative emotions can help make it less likely that you will suffer from poor sleep. Relaxation techniques can be useful for many, but if you persistently struggle with low mood, it's important to discuss this with your doctor.

Mood and sleep

An anxious mood triggers an arousal in the body that makes sleep challenging. More positive emotions can trigger the same stress response, but we are less likely to perceive it as a problem.

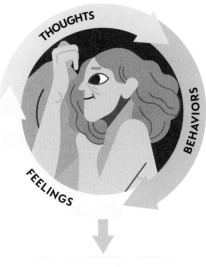

THOUGHTS

BEHAVIORS

FEELINGS

Mood
Thoughts, feelings, and behaviors combine to determine emotional state.

Positive feelings
- Excited
- Happy
- Relaxed

Negative feelings
- Worried
- Anxious
- Angry

Good night's sleep
A relaxed mood translates to a relaxed body and a peaceful night's rest.

Disrupted sleep
An aroused nervous system may cause disturbed sleep—whether it was caused by "positive" or "negative" feelings.

"Normal" state

You have no worries about sleep; when bedtime comes, you fall asleep easily.

7 p.m.:
No negative thoughts about sleep

10:30 p.m.:
Go to bed and fall asleep

Unconditioned response:
Normal sleep

Trigger for sleeplessness

You don't worry about sleep, but once in bed, you are awakened or kept awake by something.

7 p.m.:
No negative thoughts about sleep

10:30 p.m.:
Go to bed—trigger (such as outside noise) occurs

Sleeplessness or disturbed sleep

Anxiety develops

Once a trigger has interfered with sleep, you begin to worry about going to bed.

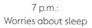

Will I sleep tonight?

7 p.m.:
Worries about sleep

10:30 p.m.:
Go to bed worried you won't sleep

Sleeplessness

Conditioned arousal

Worrying starts earlier and becomes more severe, repeatedly keeping you awake.

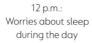

I'm dreading bedtime

12 p.m.:
Worries about sleep during the day

10:30 p.m.:
Go to bed; worries escalate

Chronic sleeplessness

Why does the thought of going to bed make me anxious?

It's a strange and intensely frustrating experience; only half an hour ago, you felt ready for sleep, but as you get ready for bed, you've become increasingly worried that you won't be able to sleep.

Many of us know the feeling of falling or being asleep, then suddenly being catapulted back into wakefulness. After a few nights of this, you start to worry about whether you will be able to get to sleep at all, and suddenly there's a real problem: your brain has begun to associate the idea of going to bed not with sleepiness, but with being awake, resulting in a bout of insomnia (see pages 198–199).

This phenomenon is known as "conditioned arousal," where a trigger—such as something in your sleep environment/routine—leads directly to a fear of going to bed and being unable to sleep, and this fear will further prevent or disrupt sleep. In order to break this cycle, you must retrain the brain to reassociate your bed and bedtime with relaxation and sleep instead of worry and wakefulness.

BREAKING THE NEGATIVE ASSOCIATION

By using CBTI (see pages 132–133), you can effectively learn to de-condition the association between going to bed and poor sleep. These techniques will also help remind you that you have previously slept without a problem, challenging any negative thoughts that tell you you'll never be able to sleep again.

You can also try keeping a notebook by your bed to jot down negative thoughts or worries about sleep—the act of writing effectively empties the thoughts from your mind, allowing you to drift off to sleep.

Conditioned arousal

Before conditioning, you go to bed and fall asleep normally. But once something triggers a night or two of broken sleep, the risk is that your worrying about bedtime—and the sleep problems this causes—escalate until you expect not to be able to sleep.

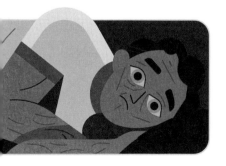

Can probiotics help with sleep?

Our gut microbiome—the naturally occurring bacteria found in our digestive tract—plays an important role in our overall health and well-being. Keeping it in peak condition could even be helpful for sleep.

Research has shown that any alterations to the gut's delicate balance of microorganisms—which can be triggered by external factors such as diet, illness, stress, and certain medications—can impact our physical and mental health.

So far, research into whether the gut microbiome can influence sleep has yielded conflicting results. One recent study found that people with a more diverse range of gut bacteria slept for longer than those with a depleted gut microbiome. A healthy gut microbiome may also be essential for those bodily processes that help regulate sleep—both serotonin and gamma-aminobutyric acid (GABA) are synthesized in the gut.

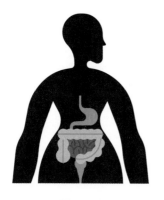

The gut

Around **90%** of the body's serotonin production occurs in the gut. Serotonin is vital for making melatonin, the sleepiness hormone.

Prebiotics

Probiotics

Better sleep

SUPPORTING YOUR GUT MICROBIOME

Eating or drinking probiotics—live bacterial cultures—will boost the diversity of your gut microbiome, which is especially helpful if you've recently taken a course of antibiotics. Probiotics are found in live yogurt and in fermented foods such as kimchi, miso, kefir, and kombucha; they can also be taken as supplements. As well as probiotics, you can support your gut health with a balanced diet and by eating foods that contain prebiotics. These are compounds that feed the gut microbiome, aiding the natural growth of beneficial bacteria. Foods rich in prebiotics include bananas, onions, garlic, oats, lentils, peas, chickpeas, beans, and peanuts.

" " _____

Growing evidence
suggests that taking steps
to improve your gut
microbiome can influence
sleep quality.

Why am I not sleepy at bedtime, even though I'm exhausted?

In the world of sleep science, "tired" and "sleepy" are very different things. Although you might feel drained at the end of the day, you won't fall asleep until that overpowering urge to drop off comes over you.

"Tiredness" is what you experience when you feel physically and mentally fatigued, whereas "sleepiness" is the irresistible desire to fall asleep. This sleep pressure (also called sleep drive or sleep urge) should increase steadily through the evening, but a range of factors can interfere. If you are always busy, you may be too awash with the stress hormones adrenaline and cortisol for the sleepiness hormone, adenosine, to increase your biological sleep pressure. Stimulants such as caffeine and certain medications can also prevent sleep pressure from building.

At the end of a busy day, we need to give ourselves adequate time to wind down, allow sleep pressure to build naturally, and make sure we can recognize the physical signs of our sleepiness.

PAST YOUR BEDTIME

Nodding off and a heaviness in your limbs are sure signs that your body is ready to fall asleep. If you don't experience these at your regular bedtime, try staying up until you are really struggling to stay awake. Doing this will let the sleep pressure build, allowing you to rediscover what it's like to feel sleepy.

Building the pressure

Ideally, your urge to sleep would follow a daily pattern like this, with sleep pressure at its lowest when you wake refreshed in the morning, then building steadily to a peak in the late evening, when you fall asleep.

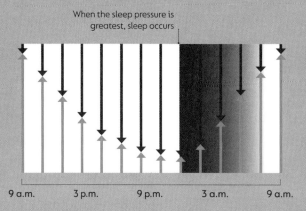

When the sleep pressure is greatest, sleep occurs

9 a.m.   3 p.m.   9 p.m.   3 a.m.   9 a.m.

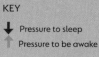

KEY

↓ Pressure to sleep

↑ Pressure to be awake

What is ASMR, and will it help me sleep?

Autonomous sensory meridian response (ASMR) describes a pleasurable sensation in the body that leaves some people physically and mentally relaxed. Many proponents say that triggering this feeling helps them sleep better.

ASMR has been described as a "braingasm": a euphoric feeling that begins with a tingling in the scalp that travels down the neck and back. This sensation is specific to ASMR, but not everyone who tries to elicit it will succeed. To date, there have been no conclusive studies into the prevalence of ASMR capability.

ASMR is, however, increasingly popular, and a whole genre of online videos has sprung up, featuring people using everyday objects to create visuals and sounds that they claim will trigger ASMR. Watching someone gently perform these rituals can be surprisingly intimate. It's this connection with the person in the video that some researchers believe triggers the release of a cocktail of pleasure- and relaxation-inducing hormones, which in turn leads to the characteristic ASMR tingle. Another suggestion is that ASMR mimics the positive bonding process between a parent and their child, resulting in a comfortable, sleep-inducing contentment.

Research on ASMR is new, but due to its reported positive effects, researchers are eager to learn more. Interestingly, although many users report that this content is deeply calming, for some, it has exactly the opposite effect; clearly, much more investigation is needed.

To see if you can experience ASMR, sit in a quiet place and watch your chosen content using headphones, focusing on how it makes you feel. You may respond more to one type of content than another, so it may be worth trying several different types of sounds and visuals.

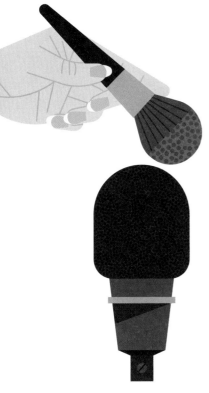

ASMR triggers

Videos often contain repeated gentle sounds, such as stroking a brush on a microphone, whispering, or crinkling paper. They may also show activities such as massage or even people eating!

Why do I fall asleep on the couch, but then as soon as I go to bed, I'm wide awake?

You're dozing off, so you go to bed. But as your head hits the pillow, sleepiness abandons you. It's frustrating, but it makes perfect sense from an evolutionary perspective. Over millions of years, our brains have evolved survival mechanisms, shifting between different states of alertness in response to our environment. The upper brain—the prefrontal cortex—is logical and strategic. Your lower brain—the limbic system—is the primitive, emotional center, and if it perceives a threat, it overrides the upper brain to trigger the "fight-or-flight" stress response to help us react to protect ourselves.

For our prehistoric ancestors, sleep was risky, leaving them vulnerable to predators. The human brain therefore developed the habit of performing a last-minute scan of surroundings to ensure it was safe to go to sleep. For modern humans, having trouble sleeping or being startled awake—even once—can lead to a situation where the act of going to bed triggers our survival instincts and readies the body to respond to lurking danger.

Time for bed
Relaxing on the couch, your watchful limbic system is deactivated and sleep comes all too easily. Once you move to the bedroom, your brain remembers there could be danger waiting—sounding the alarm and jolting you into alertness.

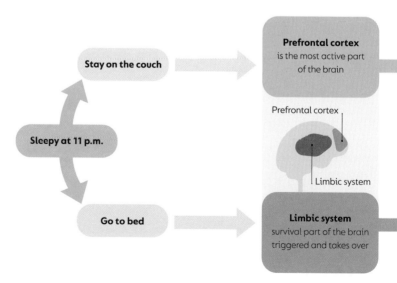

Sleepy at 11 p.m.

Stay on the couch

Go to bed

Prefrontal cortex is the most active part of the brain

Prefrontal cortex

Limbic system

Limbic system survival part of the brain triggered and takes over

SWITCHING OFF THE PRIMAL BRAIN

To overcome your primal instincts, you need to find ways to pacify the limbic system, helping your brain override its natural response to threats and reassure it that there is nothing to fear from going to bed.

• **A relaxation exercise**, such as the one on page 125, can help calm the limbic brain's state of watchfulness.

• **Does your bedroom evoke a sense of calm and security?** See pages 170–171 and 178–179 for ways to make your sleeping space feel relaxing and safe.

• **If you can, avoid situations that might trigger stress**, such as difficult conversations with a partner or family member or looking at work emails.

• **CBTI or other cognitive strategies** (see pages 132–133), which change how you perceive sleep, can be useful.

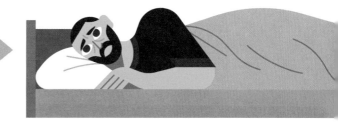

Logical brain in charge
• No threat perceived—brain feels relaxed and safe
• No stress response triggered—you stay sleepy and doze off

Primal brain in charge
• Brain, recalling previous times it was startled into wakefulness, orders scan of surroundings to check for danger
• Stress response triggered—you feel wide awake

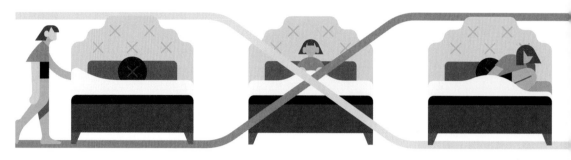

Sleepy and relaxed ...
GABA is high, cortisol low

Problems mount—cortisol rises

Feeling restless—get up

Why do my problems seem amplified at night?

Often it's while we are lying awake in bed that our problems suddenly slide into hyperfocus. As the worries intensify, the more likely they are to chase away sleep. Humans are both social creatures and solution-focused beings. If we encounter a problem during the day, we can take practical steps to solve it or reach out to others for help. At night, with no distractions and no one to discuss our problems with, the brain seizes the opportunity to turn minor worries into major complications. Lying in the dark, you slip into catastrophic thinking—conjuring up worst-case scenarios and feeling increasingly helpless. This can trigger your body's stress response, flooding your system with adrenaline and cortisol and sending your nervous system into overdrive.

CALMING YOUR STRESS RESPONSE

One simple, proven way to counter this stress response is to move. Movement requires conscious action, so it gives you a sense of taking control of your problems. In addition, studies have shown that movement increases levels of gamma-aminobutyric acid (GABA). GABA is a neurotransmitter naturally produced by the body that

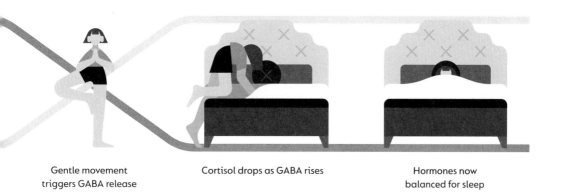

Gentle movement
triggers GABA release

Cortisol drops as GABA rises

Hormones now
balanced for sleep

slows activity in the nervous system, calming the stress
response and neutralizing any associated negative
feelings. Stress can inhibit GABA production, and low
levels of GABA are linked to anxiety and poor sleep, so
boosting GABA at bedtime could be enough to banish
your worries and help you get to sleep.

Try making gentle movement part of your relaxation
routine before bed. Yoga in particular has been shown
to lead to a notable increase in GABA. If you find your
problems are still going around in your head after 20
minutes in bed, try getting up again and undertaking
some gentle movement to trigger GABA release.

SUPPLEMENTING GABA

There's some evidence to suggest that taking a GABA
supplement, or the natural herbal remedy ashwagandha
(which has GABA-like properties), can also reduce stress
and aid sleep. Interestingly, probiotic and fermented foods
such as kefir or kimchi can promote GABA production in
the gut, so adding these foods to your diet may also help
promote healthy levels of GABA.

KEY

GABA level
Cortisol level

GABA and cortisol

When our problems become
amplified, the body's stress response
is activated, which decreases GABA.
Triggering a release of GABA sends
cortisol down again, paving the way
back to restful sleep.

What should I do if I can't get back to sleep?

Most of us wake at one time or another during the night—possibly to visit the bathroom or to change position—but getting back to sleep can be a challenge for some.

It's not unusual to wake in the night, and most people will quickly fall back to sleep naturally, or possibly with the help of some music, a sleep app, or a few pages of a book. However, if you haven't fallen asleep after 20 minutes and are lying in bed tossing and turning, the best strategy is to get up and leave your bedroom for a short time until you feel sleepy again.

DISTRACT YOURSELF

Getting out of bed may seem counterintuitive, but trying to will yourself back to sleep is not only futile, but can also trigger more long-term sleep problems, such as insomnia, as those niggling worries about not being able to sleep start to creep in. In addition, when we can't sleep, we tend to try hard not to move, which creates tension in the body, pushing sleep farther from our reach. Evidence shows that getting up and doing something else is the best way to tackle this issue. Ultimately, sleep is about relaxation, not trying hard. If this affects you regularly, plan ahead by preparing a toolkit of distractions. These should be pleasurable but not too stimulating—maybe an undemanding book, some adult coloring, or a relaxing stretching or yoga routine.

Keep lights low and when you start to feel sleepy, go back to bed. If sleep doesn't come after another 20 minutes, get up and try this low-key distraction method again.

" " _____

Trying hard to sleep is
counterproductive, so
stop and do something
else to help your natural
sleepiness return.

Why can't I remember my dreams?

Everybody dreams, but not everyone remembers what they dreamt. The ability to recall a dream seems to depend on many factors, including the stage of sleep from which you wake.

Research suggests that there are certain conditions required in order for us to remember dreams, and if these are not met, the dream simply slips away before we wake. These factors include how notable a dream is, the length of time between the dream and waking, the stage in your sleep cycle at which you wake, and events immediately after waking.

Some scientists have also theorized that the ability to remember a dream is linked to being left-handed. In left-handed people, the right hemisphere of the brain is

Dream recall theory

Some sleep scientists have theorized that a specific set of conditions determine whether or not we remember a dream.

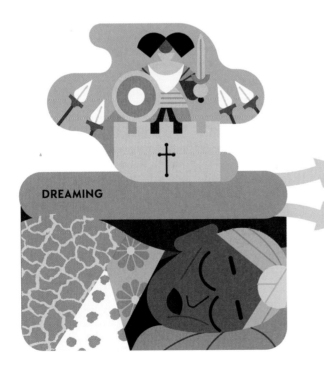

DREAMING

GOOD RECALL CONDITIONS

- Exciting dream content
- Waking from REM sleep
- Waking soon after the dream
- No disruption before the dream is transferred to long-term memory

POOR RECALL CONDITIONS

- Boring, uneventful dream
- Waking from a non-REM sleep stage
- Waking too long after the dream
- Interrupted before the dream content is stored in long-term memory (for example, alarm clock goes off)

larger. As this is the area in which dreams are formed, it's possible that left-handers might dream more and have better access to their dreams for recall. Studies have shown that left-handers also experience more REM sleep—the stage during which the majority of dreaming takes place.

TEENAGE DREAMS

The amount of REM sleep we get appears to play a major role in remembering dreams. Teenagers clock up the most REM sleep and also have the best dream recall of any age group. As we age, both REM sleep and dream recollection diminish.

HOW TO REMEMBER YOUR DREAMS

- **Get between seven** and nine hours of sleep to ensure maximum REM sleep, which increases the potential for dreaming and dream recall.

- **Keep a dream journal** by your bed and, before you fall asleep, remind yourself that you want to remember your dreams. When you wake, fragments of your dreams will be stored in your short-term memory, so write them down quickly before they are wiped. Repeatedly capturing dreams on paper has been shown to enhance dream recall.

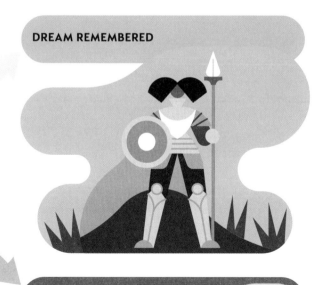

DREAM REMEMBERED

DREAM FORGOTTEN

80–90%

of dreams are remembered
when waking from REM sleep.
For sleep Stages 1 and 2,
the chance of recall
is less than 50%,
and for Stage-3
deep sleep, it's 0%

Why are my dreams more vivid when I'm stressed?

Stress and anxiety can leave us sleep deprived and short on REM sleep. This means that the next time we sleep, we fall into REM more quickly and remain in it for longer, something known as "REM rebound."

Although we can dream in both REM and non-REM sleep, research shows that REM dreams tend to be in vivid technicolor and have bizarre content, whereas non-REM dreams are slower, more conceptual, and usually in black and white. This might be because during REM-sleep dreams, the hypothalamus, the brain's emotional center, is extremely active, whereas the prefrontal cortex, the brain's logical region, is less active. Therefore, when we spend more time in REM sleep, as we do when we are stressed, our dreams may in fact be more surreal and evocative than usual.

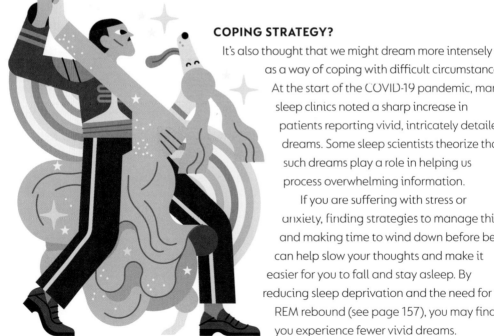

COPING STRATEGY?

It's also thought that we might dream more intensely as a way of coping with difficult circumstances. At the start of the COVID-19 pandemic, many sleep clinics noted a sharp increase in patients reporting vivid, intricately detailed dreams. Some sleep scientists theorize that such dreams play a role in helping us process overwhelming information.

If you are suffering with stress or anxiety, finding strategies to manage this and making time to wind down before bed can help slow your thoughts and make it easier for you to fall and stay asleep. By reducing sleep deprivation and the need for REM rebound (see page 157), you may find you experience fewer vivid dreams.

Why are my dreams so scary?

Waking from a nightmare can upset you mentally and physically, leaving you with a niggling sense of unease throughout the day.

We all have bad dreams from time to time, but sleep scientists define a nightmare as a dream that evokes unpleasant emotions and physical sensations that are powerful enough to wake you.

The themes of nightmares are surprisingly similar among different groups; the most common include teeth falling out, being chased or attacked, the death of a loved one, or being paralyzed. Underlying stress, anxiety, or depression are often the trigger for adult nightmares; fragments of real-life experiences or worries combine with random content to create terrifying dreams. People living with posttraumatic stress disorder (PTSD) are especially vulnerable to recurrent, repetitive nightmares.

" "
A US study found that 52% of war veterans suffered regular nightmares compared to just 3% of civilians.

SURVIVAL MECHANISM

The "threat simulation" theory of dreaming suggests that scary dreams are an evolved defense mechanism. As we dream, by rehearsing our responses to dangerous situations and strengthening the neural pathways required for us to be alert, we increase our chances of survival in the waking world. This could explain why those who live in unsafe environments, such as a war zone, tend to report more nightmares.

If nightmares become regular and impact both your sleeping and waking life, don't suffer alone: seek your doctor's advice. A variety of factors could be driving this, and an appropriate course of "talking" treatment and/or medication can be very effective in breaking the pattern.

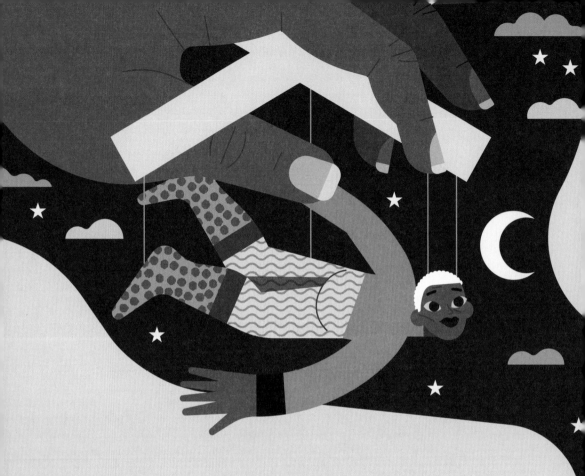

Can I learn to lucid dream?

Imagine having a dream where you could choose your actions. It might take practice, but the ability to control our dreams is thought to be something we all have the potential to do.

Lucid dreaming, where the dreamer is aware they are dreaming, is not uncommon—it's thought that around 20 percent of people have at least one lucid dream a month. In such a dream, you are asleep, but your mind believes you are conscious, so your prefrontal cortex—the part of your brain responsible for decision-making—is active in the same way it would be if you were awake. So dreamers have the potential to be able to actively shape their dream content and could feasibly use their dreams to hone skills, find a solution to a problem, or take control and bring a nightmare to an end.

MASTERING THE TECHNIQUE

This is a relatively new area of investigation in sleep research, but several studies have found that lucid dreamers are able to change the setting or deliberately wake themselves from a dream. Scientists have developed techniques to help dreamers recognize when they are dreaming, although results so far are inconsistent. The findings indicate that learning to lucid dream takes practice, and even then it isn't possible for everyone.

To try it, start by telling yourself you are going to dream that night. Keep a dream journal by your bed and jot down any dreams as soon as you wake. By monitoring your dreams, you can work up to being aware of them and possibly even directing them. Make sure you get enough sleep; REM is where the majority of dreaming takes place, so being short on sleep means missed opportunities to lucid dream.

DREAM YOGA

Tibetan Buddhists have practiced lucid dreaming— they call it dream yoga— for more than 2,000 years. An advanced meditation technique, practitioners use it to gain insight into their emotional state, provide inner clarity of thought, and deepen spirituality.

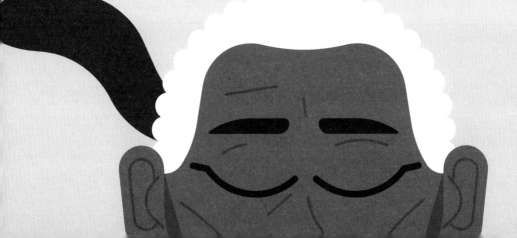

Why do I get my most creative ideas while dozing off or sleeping?

Sleep is rich in creative potential. While we sleep, our intuitive brain has the opportunity to make novel associations and connections—resulting in new ideas upon waking.

Throughout the course of the day, so many ideas float in and out of our minds that we don't always get a chance to give them the attention they deserve. When sleep rolls around, you finally relax and new connections in the brain occur.

HYPNOGOGIC CREATIVITY

As the body transitions from wakefulness to sleep, the brain, too, is in flux. This liminal in-between state where you are just beginning to dream but are still conscious is known as the hypnogogic state and can result in sensory hallucinations. The exact cause has long been unknown, but research suggests that during this state, we produce both alpha and theta brainwaves. Under normal sleep conditions, these two states don't occur at the same time, and it may be the brief combination of both that gives

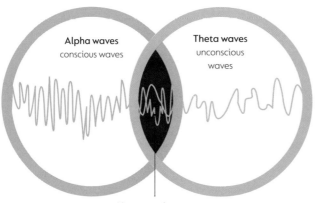

Alpha waves
conscious waves

Theta waves
unconscious waves

Hypnogogic state
both brainwaves occur
simultaneously

Combination of waves
During the hypnogogic state, resting alpha waves associated with conscious relaxation and slow theta waves associated with unconsciousness briefly occur together.

rise to visions and physical sensations. Scientists have also observed that in the hypnogogic state, there is less activity in the prefrontal cortex, the seat of logical thinking. This may lead to more intuitive thinking, which could trigger bursts of creativity.

DREAM BIG

We are also creative during REM sleep, which is the stage where we do most of our dreaming. REM sleep is dominated by two types of brain waves: theta, the slow waves associated with memory and learning, and beta, which is faster and similar to brain activity when we are awake. Also, the areas of our brain responsible for sensory and emotional information are especially active, which can lead to creative and artistic idea generation.

There have been many instances of musicians, scientists, and authors who have had their biggest and best ideas while dreaming. Paul McCartney, The Rolling Stones, and Billy Joel all claim to have had songs, melodies, and lyrics come to them while dreaming; and the creator of the periodic table of elements, Dmitri Mendeleev, wrote that the complete table first appeared to him in a dream.

To recall what you discovered in these bursts of creative dreaming, you need to write down or record dreams as soon as you wake; they will disappear from your short-term memory very soon after waking.

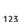

How do I stop my mind racing so I can sleep?

Sometimes the speed at which our thoughts race through our mind can be overwhelming and leave us lying awake at night. For sleep to come, we must find a way to switch our brains from a state of high alert to deep relaxation. The key to slowing your brain activity at night and allowing your mind to empty is not necessarily to try to banish your thoughts, but rather to allow them to be present without being consumed or overwhelmed by them.

Mindfulness is a scientifically validated way to manage emotions and mental health that has its roots in the ancient practices of Buddhism. It is the act of becoming fully present with what is happening in the here and now without judgment. By focusing the mind in this way, we are able to put the brakes on our procession of thoughts.

Physiologically, mindfulness enables us to slow the speed of brainwaves. Fast brainwaves facilitate problem-solving and alertness, whereas slower waves allow for more time between thoughts, which helps us untangle ourselves from their overwhelming effects.

Meditation is another practice that can be effective in slowing thoughts. It often uses breathing techniques in conjunction with mindfulness to bring a greater awareness to the present moment.

Brainwave range

We constantly move between four different brainwave states, depending on whether or not we are awake and how active or relaxed the mind is.

Beta brainwaves
Awake; alert; engaged in conscious thought.

Alpha brainwaves
Conscious but physically and mentally relaxed.

Theta brainwaves
Reduced consciousness; able to dream; creativity high.

5, 4, 3, 2, 1 mindfulness

Take a moment to breathe deeply: in through your nose for a count of five, then out through your mouth for a count of seven. Then work through the steps, paying attention only to the task in hand without passing judgment.

There are many different ways to use mindfulness and meditation, with excellent apps, books, and podcasts to guide you. Some practices are designed to slow you down before bed, while others help you fall back asleep if you wake with a racing mind. Many people try meditation for the first time before bed, only to give up because it doesn't seem to work. Meditation takes time to master: the trick is to practice during the day so that when you actually need it, you have a tried-and-true relaxation tool to draw on.

The mindfulness exercise on this page can help you ground your thoughts in the present. Try repeating the exercise until you feel that your thoughts are sufficiently slowed to enable rest.

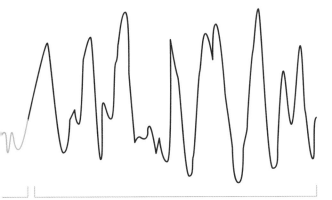

Delta brainwaves
Unconscious; in a deep, dreamless, and restorative sleep.

5 things you can see:
such as your hands, the room around you, a picture, your dog in his bed, a bedside lamp.

4 things you can feel:
such as your nightclothes, mattress springs, the weight of your cover, a breeze on your face.

3 things you can hear:
such as your breath, the hum of traffic, the creak of the central heating.

2 things you can smell:
such as soap, bed linens.

1 thing you can taste:
such as your toothpaste.

Does counting sheep really work?

Visualizing and counting sheep to bring on sleep is common across many cultures, but science shows that this strategy is unlikely to be very effective.

The idea of counting sheep to aid sleepiness may have stemmed from the fact that historically, shepherds had to tally up their flock at night before they could relax and go to sleep. While it's true that focusing the mind on a mental task may distract you from any worries that might be keeping you awake, it's more likely that counting sheep will leave you feeling restless and bored rather than drowsy—and there's a good reason for this.

For people suffering with insomnia or who struggle to fall asleep due to racing thoughts, counting sheep is so simple and repetitive that the brain is not sufficiently engaged in the task to distract you from your worries or to tire you out.

Research shows that exercises that are interesting, engaging, and image-based lead to a quicker sleep onset, as these activities keep the mind busy enough to distract it from other thoughts until it has expended enough energy to make it ready for sleep. Instead of sheep auditing, try the guided imagery exercise on pages 128–129.

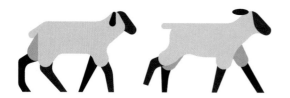
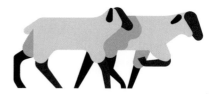

" " _____

A study of people with
insomnia found that
performing boring mental
tasks resulted in them
taking longer to fall asleep.

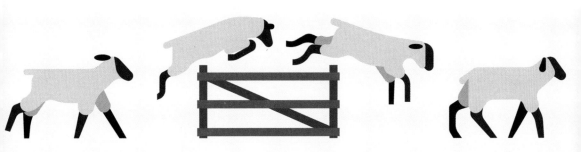

I regularly wake at 3 a.m.—how can I get back to sleep?

Waking during the night is normal and very common—and around 3 a.m. is the time that people most often find themselves wide awake. The key to drifting back off is to stay calm and relaxed.

Assuming an 11 p.m. bedtime, around 3 a.m. marks the transition from deep sleep to longer periods of REM. As the brain is more active in this stage, it's more likely that you'll wake. Also, by the early hours, you have used up most of the sleep pressure that helped you get to sleep. Levels of the sleepiness hormone melatonin dip as production starts up of hormones that will help you wake up. These factors can all lead to early-hours wakefulness.

Once awake, it's all too easy to focus on the fact that you aren't asleep—for instance, by clock watching—and this tends to make the situation worse. The body's stress response is triggered, and the resulting spike of cortisol catapults us into a fully awake state.

Lying awake at 3 a.m. can feel very lonely, so finding tools to help is essential. One proven technique is using guided imagery: by visualizing something pleasurable, this keeps mind and body calm, avoiding the release of stress hormones. Research shows that people who practice guided imagery fall back to sleep more quickly than those who don't. If this issue affects you, try the exercise on the opposite page. As with all such techniques, it gets easier with practice, so stick with it for best results.

AVOID SUGAR LOWS

Waking at night is sometimes due to blood sugar dipping in the small hours. This condition is known as nocturnal hypoglycemia, and it is also a common cause of insomnia. If you suspect this might be causing your waking, try a small snack, such as a few crackers, just before bed. Avoid fatty, spicy, or processed foods so as not to stress your digestive system.

GUIDED IMAGERY

Practice this exercise during the day when you are not anxious so you will know how to do it when the need arises. Slowly work through the steps, keeping your focus only on your breath and the sensations you are imagining.

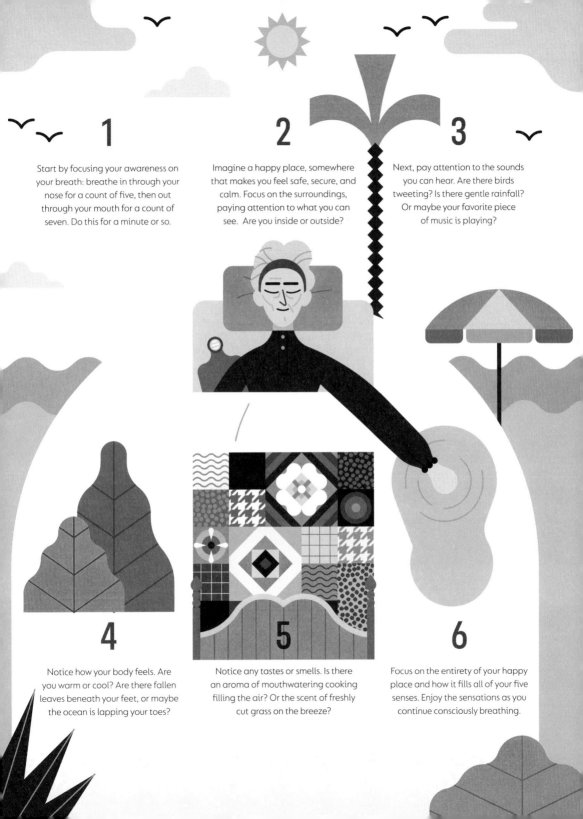

1

Start by focusing your awareness on your breath: breathe in through your nose for a count of five, then out through your mouth for a count of seven. Do this for a minute or so.

2

Imagine a happy place, somewhere that makes you feel safe, secure, and calm. Focus on the surroundings, paying attention to what you can see. Are you inside or outside?

3

Next, pay attention to the sounds you can hear. Are there birds tweeting? Is there gentle rainfall? Or maybe your favorite piece of music is playing?

4

Notice how your body feels. Are you warm or cool? Are there fallen leaves beneath your feet, or maybe the ocean is lapping your toes?

5

Notice any tastes or smells. Is there an aroma of mouthwatering cooking filling the air? Or the scent of freshly cut grass on the breeze?

6

Focus on the entirety of your happy place and how it fills all of your five senses. Enjoy the sensations as you continue consciously breathing.

How do anxiety and depression affect sleep?

We all feel low or worried at times, but anxiety and depression are chronic disorders that have a negative relationship with sleep: both cause sleep disruptions, and, in turn, sleep problems exacerbate these conditions. When worry or fear has become excessive and difficult to control, it can be termed anxiety. Constant fretting may keep a person awake at night, and the dread of something bad happening also triggers the body's stress response, keeping it in a state of alertness and preventing sleep. To compound the situation, after a bad night's sleep, a person with anxiety may worry this will happen again, reinforcing the idea that going to bed means sleeplessness, which perpetuates the cycle of poor sleep and often leads to insomnia (see pages 104–105).

Similarly, a person with chronically poor sleep may develop a "fear" of sleep, which can trigger worry that extends to other areas of life, resulting in an anxiety condition. One study found that a single night of sleeplessness can increase anxiety levels by up to 30 percent, and conversely that sufficient deep sleep helps reduce anxiety.

Feeling anxious > Can't sleep > Wake up tired > Worry about going to sleep > Develop a fear of going to sleep > Can't sleep

Anxiety increases

DEPRESSION

Depression is a mood disorder that interferes with a person's ability to manage daily life. People often experience a sense of hopelessness, poor concentration, and reduced appetite, as well as feeling tired during the day and sleeping badly at night. Up to 90 percent of people with depression report problems with their sleep, and it seems clear that hormone imbalances are at least partly responsible. Serotonin, the "happiness" hormone, plays a key role in producing melatonin. Because depression is associated with low levels of serotonin, it is not surprising that sleep problems are so common among those with depression.

Some evidence suggests that people with depression spend more time in REM sleep than other stages, meaning that they miss out on the deep sleep necessary for rest and repair, and they don't feel refreshed when they wake. This can lead to a further lowering of mood and a cycle of poor sleep and depression. Research is ongoing to ascertain whether reducing REM sleep would be effective in treating depression and improving sleep quality.

BREAKING THE CYCLE

Addressing the underlying factors that maintain anxiety and depression is the best strategy for dealing with poor sleep associated with these conditions, and it's important to speak to your doctor to discuss therapeutic support and medication options—more studies are underway and treatments are advancing all the time.

Self-help techniques measurably improve things for many; relaxation strategies (see pages 80–81) and distraction techniques (see pages 124–125) can help you switch off or slow racing thoughts, and CBTI (see pages 132–133) is extremely useful for identifying and challenging entrenched thoughts and feelings that might be compounding your sleep issues.

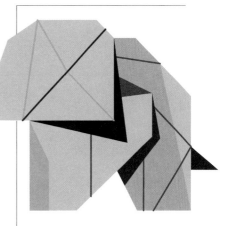

CALM WITH CREATIVITY

Research has convincingly shown that creative activities such as model making, origami, coloring, or even building with toy bricks can all trigger a calming response that helps combat anxiety. Because they require both mental concentration and physical dexterity, these activities shift your focus and allow your brain to enter a more meditative state and become less focused on troubling thoughts.

Can CBTI help me sleep?

If you have trouble sleeping, it's natural to worry about it, but if bedtime becomes a source of anxiety that further feeds sleeplessness, cognitive behavioral therapy for insomnia (CBTI) may help.

If you consistently experience poor sleep, sleeplessness may become a self-fulfilling prophecy—the more you believe that you will struggle to sleep, the more you worry, and this in turn increases the likelihood that you'll suffer sleep problems.

HOW CBTI WORKS

Ideally, thinking about your bed and going to sleep would stimulate a positive response from you rather than one of dread. CBTI works by improving your relationship with sleep, helping you change the negative thoughts, feelings, and behaviors associated with going to bed that have become the very things that keep you awake.

There are five aspects of CBTI, each undertaken simultaneously (see opposite page). This approach has proved highly effective in moving patients from a position of frustratedly trying to force themselves to sleep to calmly allowing sleep to happen. Once a sleep problem is overcome, if it starts to become an issue again, patients can reintroduce the CBTI techniques they have learned to prevent the problem from escalating.

It's relatively easy to access CBTI; you can discuss options with your doctor or find a qualified sleep therapist yourself. Treatment by trained professionals is offered individually or in a group. You can also undertake self-guided treatment via a range of effective apps, online courses, or books.

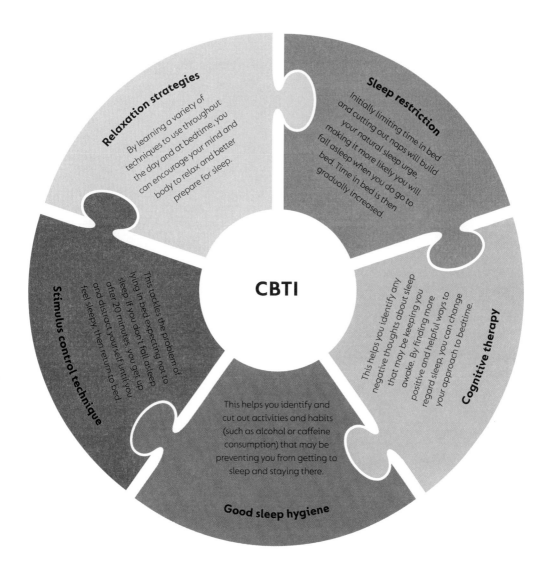

Relaxation strategies
By learning a variety of techniques to use throughout the day and at bedtime, you can encourage your mind and body to relax and better prepare for sleep.

Sleep restriction
Initially limiting time in bed and cutting out naps will build your natural sleep urge, making it more likely you will fall asleep when you do go to bed. Time in bed is then gradually increased.

CBTI

Stimulus control technique
This tackles the problem of lying in bed expecting not to sleep. If you don't fall asleep after 20 minutes, you get up and distract yourself until you feel sleepy, then return to bed.

Cognitive therapy
This helps you identify any negative thoughts about sleep that may be keeping you awake. By finding you positive and helpful ways to regard sleep, you can change your approach to bedtime.

This helps you identify and cut out activities and habits (such as alcohol or caffeine consumption) that may be preventing you from getting to sleep and staying there.

Good sleep hygiene

The CBTI toolkit
CBTI helps break negative associations between bedtime and sleeplessness by taking an integrated approach made up of five linked components and strategies.

How can hypnotherapy help with sleep?

There is a growing body of evidence that hypnosis can be used therapeutically to reduce insomnia and to improve conditions that impact negatively on sleep, such as anxiety and irritable bowel syndrome.

The Greek word "hypnos" translates as "sleep," but during hypnosis, you are not actually asleep. You are conscious of your surroundings, while your body is in deep relaxation and brain activity slows right down. Think about how you feel just at the moment of falling asleep—this is the "theta state," during which the brain generates very slow, high-amplitude theta waves. This is very different from the state you experience during meditation, in which the brain produces medium-speed, relaxed-but-alert alpha waves.

WHAT TO EXPECT

Hypnosis should always be delivered by a qualified professional who is preferably an expert in sleep issues. During a session, your therapist will bring you to a relaxed state using verbal cues (certain words or phrases), by directing your focus to an object, or a combination of both. They will then gently suggest ways to change your perceptions and habits around sleep. Because you are in a slower-wave brain state, you absorb these suggestions on a deeper level, making you more able to act on these once you return to normal consciousness.

Around 10 percent of patients are deemed by practitioners as "highly hypnotizable," while for roughly the same percentage, hypnosis won't work at all. Most of us fall somewhere between the two extremes, and there is no doubt that for many with sleep issues, this therapy can be effective and beneficial. If you have a specific sleep issue, it's worth seeking out a therapist to discuss whether hypnotherapy could be appropriate for you.

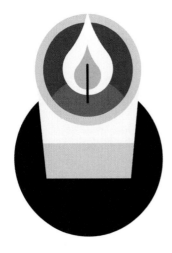

" " ——————————

Hypnotherapy can help patients increase the time they spend in slow-wave, restorative sleep by as much as **80%**.

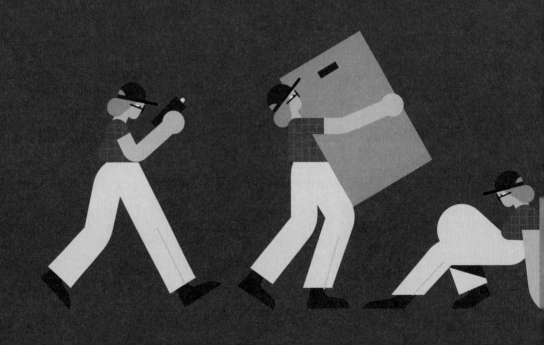

Lifestyle

Your daily routine, work commitments, and personal preferences all play a role in what happens once you close your eyes at the end of the day. By understanding what helps and hinders sleep, you can make the best choices to help you get the rest you need.

Are naps harmful or helpful?

To nap or not to nap? Whether napping will work for you depends on a range of factors, such as lifestyle; sleep cycle length; culture; and, most importantly, the length of your snooze.

If you like to nap, you are not alone. Napping is part of the culture in many countries: around 51 percent of people worldwide habitually enjoy 40 winks in the daytime.

When it comes to napping, one size definitely doesn't fit all. If you are sleep deprived, a nap can be helpful or even essential for making it through the day. However, for those with other sleep issues, a nap may make it harder to fall asleep at night. For most of us, the timing and length of our nap will largely determine how beneficial it is to our sleep routine.

It's all in the timing

An ideal nap lasts one full sleep cycle—but in practice, this is hard to control. The most convenient and achievable option is a nap of 30 minutes or less, waking before the deep-sleep phase begins.

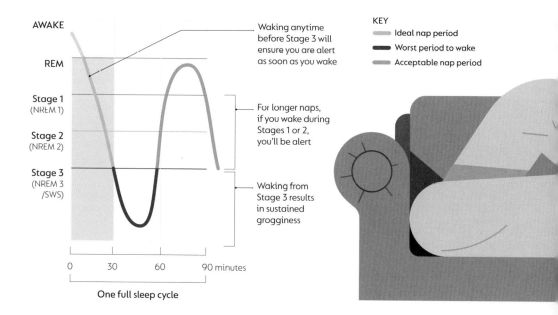

AWAKE

REM

Stage 1
(NREM 1)

Stage 2
(NREM 2)

Stage 3
(NREM 3
/SWS)

0   30   60   90 minutes

One full sleep cycle

Waking anytime before Stage 3 will ensure you are alert as soon as you wake

For longer naps, if you wake during Stages 1 or 2, you'll be alert

Waking from Stage 3 results in sustained grogginess

KEY
- Ideal nap period
- Worst period to wake
- Acceptable nap period

SHORTER IS BETTER

• **Between 1 p.m. and 4 p.m.**, most people experience an increase in sleepiness, triggered by a slight drop in core body temperature. A nap of 30 minutes or less around this time allows you to benefit from a burst of Stage 1 and 2 sleep, which is good for mental and physical alertness.

• **Napping for 30 minutes or less** can reduce stress and lower the risk of cardiovascular problems like heart attacks and strokes. One study showed that napping three times a week for 30 minutes led to a 37 percent decreased risk of dying from heart disease.

• **A brief nap can be beneficial** for those with excessive daytime sleepiness, including people suffering from sleep apnea or narcolepsy, shift workers, and people with jet lag. Studies show that short naps can help improve or reset a disrupted circadian rhythm.

UNHELPFUL NAPS

• Naps can interfere with insomnia treatment, which involves restricting daytime sleep to increase the likelihood of sleeping solidly at night.

• Beware of naps of more than 30 minutes. Waking from the deep-sleep stages results in sleep inertia, a super-groggy state where brainwaves are slow and it takes longer to adjust to the awake state.

• A recent study has found that napping for more than 60 minutes a day increased the risk of type 2 diabetes by 50 percent. If you are in a high-risk category for this condition, avoid regular long naps.

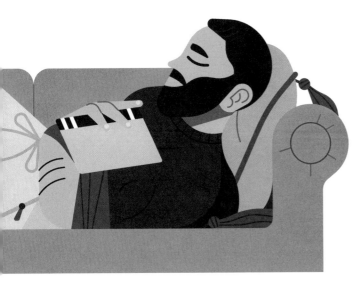

" "

A **30-minute power nap** gives an energy boost and is a healthier option than caffeine.

Is good sleep continuous, or can it come in chunks?

There's an ongoing debate as to whether or not splitting the amount of slumber you get into chunks is the key to "good sleep." Sleeping in this way has advantages for some, but it's not for everyone.

Sleeping in one stretch each night is termed "monophasic sleep" by clinicians. Biphasic sleep is where your sleep is split into two sessions with a period of wakefulness in between, and polyphasic sleep is sleep split into multiple chunks across a 24-hour period.

Most people in the West have monophasic sleep, sleeping in a single seven-to-nine-hour chunk each night, but in some regions—especially in hot climates—people tend toward biphasic sleep. For example, in Spain, stores traditionally close for a few hours after lunch so people can nap during the afternoon heat before staying up late and sleeping for a shorter time at night. Polyphasic sleep is most prevalent among people who need to be awake at random points throughout the day and night, such as new parents, but there is evidence that long-term polyphasic sleep patterns can have a negative effect on health.

TIMING YOUR SLEEP CHUNKS

If you choose a biphasic or polyphasic sleep pattern, pay attention to the length of your "sleep chunks." Less than six continuous hours of sleep generally is not long enough to complete all the sleep stages needed for optimum rest and repair. (One sleep cycle takes up to 90 minutes, and it is ideal to complete four to five cycles in one sleep session.) So a monophasic sleep pattern gives most people the best chance of achieving good, restorative sleep. However, if work or lifestyle makes it difficult to achieve this, try to ensure that one of your sleeping chunks is long enough to let your body complete its cycle of rest and repair.

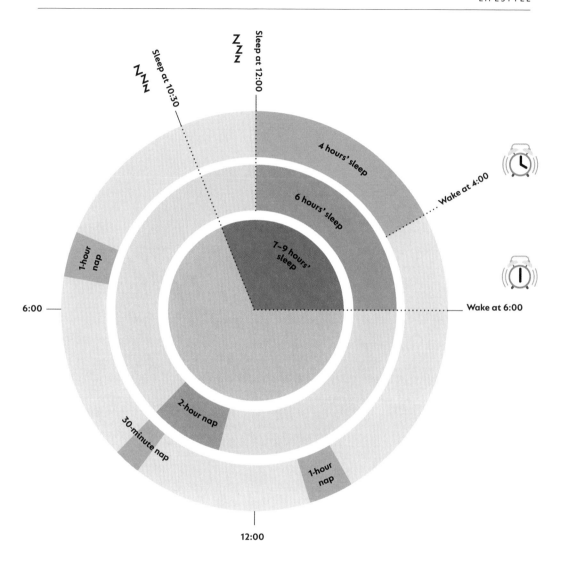

Sleep at 10:30

ZZZ

Sleep at 12:00

ZZZ

4 hours' sleep

6 hours' sleep

7–9 hours' sleep

Wake at 4:00

Wake at 6:00

1-hour nap

6:00

2-hour nap

30-minute nap

1-hour nap

12:00

Segmenting your sleep

These examples illustrate that a monophasic sleep pattern is best suited to someone with a "9 to 5" lifestyle. A biphasic pattern could include an afternoon sleep, as shown here, or any combination of two chunks of sleep.

KEY

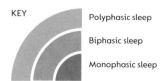

Polyphasic sleep

Biphasic sleep

Monophasic sleep

Can I catch up on sleep?

The prospect of sleeping in on the weekend is one of life's great pleasures. Going to bed, you turn off your alarm in the hope that more sleep will ease the fatigue of the week. So why do you wake up tired after you sleep in?

Catching up on sleep on the weekend may sound straightforward, but it's not quite as simple as that—there's only so much lost sleep we can recover. On average, we need around one hour of sleep for every two hours we've been awake, but hours spent in bed don't equal hours spent asleep, and a lot of us fall short of this.

When we don't achieve the sleep we need, we end up with what is known as "sleep debt." This is the gap between the amount of sleep you should get, given how long you've been awake, and the amount you do end up getting. Whenever we shave a little time off our night's sleep, the shortfall increases—the more we do it, the more debt rolls over to the next day, leaving our brains struggling to function.

We can't repay sleep debt by bingeing on sleep on the weekends, because we can only realistically recoup an extra few hours on top of our usual nightly total before it interferes with our circadian rhythms (see pages 22–23), and this isn't enough to undo the effects of the lack of sleep we've built up across the week. Trying to catch up on sleep can also leave us with headaches and feeling worse than if we hadn't attempted it—spending longer in bed means less chance to rehydrate. The best solution is to avoid sleep debt, or at least keep it to a minimum.

HOW TO AVOID SLEEP DEBT

• **Start with bedtime.** Go to bed earlier, but wake up at your normal time. This allows for more sleep each night without disrupting your body clock's natural wake time.

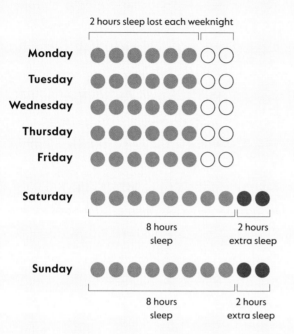

2 hours sleep lost each weeknight

Monday
Tuesday
Wednesday
Thursday
Friday

Saturday
| 8 hours sleep | 2 hours extra sleep |

Sunday
| 8 hours sleep | 2 hours extra sleep |

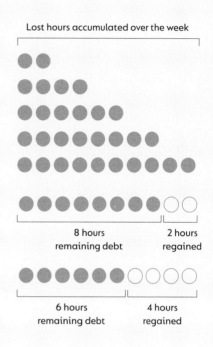

Lost hours accumulated over the week

Saturday
| 8 hours remaining debt | 2 hours regained |

Sunday
| 6 hours remaining debt | 4 hours regained |

• **Keep a sleep diary.** Track your routine over a 24-hour period for a couple of weeks to measure how much sleep you get and figure out exactly where your sleep debt is occurring. A diary will also help you identify any factors that are impacting your ability to get to bed early enough to get the sleep you need. An example of a sleep diary and how to use it can be found on pages 36–37.

• **Napping can help, but timing matters.** Napping can help offset sleep debt, but make sure you don't nap too close to bedtime, as this will make it harder to fall asleep at night and create even more sleep debt. To get the most from your nap, check out the advice on pages 138–139.

Accumulated weekly sleep debt

Falling two hours short of the sleep you need each night during the week means that, by the weekend, you will be owed 10 hours of sleep. Despite sleeping in on Saturday and Sunday, by the end of the weekend, you're still deeply in sleep debt.

Why does my body clock go haywire at times?

When your body's internal timekeeping system gets off kilter, you might find yourself napping at work, waking up hungry in the night, or feeling too hyped up to sleep. Your body clock does more than dictate sleeping and waking; it affects the daily rhythms of biological processes throughout the body, from metabolism to muscle growth. The master clock in your brain (see pages 22–23) sets the pace by sending out hormonal, chemical, body temperature, and other signals to peripheral clocks in the cells of your tissues and organs in order to synchronize their specific daily cycles so your body functions optimally.

Scientists have found that this complex circadian timing system relies on internal and external cues called "zeitgebers" ("time-givers" in German). Lifestyle factors can create conflict between clocks and upset the system—but you can also work with these cues to reset or "entrain" it.

KEY ZEITGEBERS

Natural daylight is the most important zeitgeber for sleep. It's received via cells in the eyes that constantly measure light levels and relay information to the body's master clock. The brain then increases or reduces production of melatonin, the hormone that makes you sleepy.

Food intake is a zeitgeber, because we metabolize food differently during the 24-hour cycle. Research shows that the timing of meals can shift sleep/wake times, while constant snacking can disrupt them, potentially leading to weight gain, lack of energy, and metabolic problems. Some studies suggest meal timing could be a more important cue for some peripheral clocks than light.

Because our body temperature fluctuates to mirror the sleep/wake cycle, external temperature is another zeitgeber that can affect sleep by disrupting this cycle.

SLEEP AND COVID-19

For many people, not having to commute during lockdowns offered an opportunity to reset their circadian rhythm and pay off their sleep "debt." For others, the loss of routine for eating, exercise, and time outdoors meant inconsistent zeitgebers and disrupted body clocks—resulting in poorer sleep.

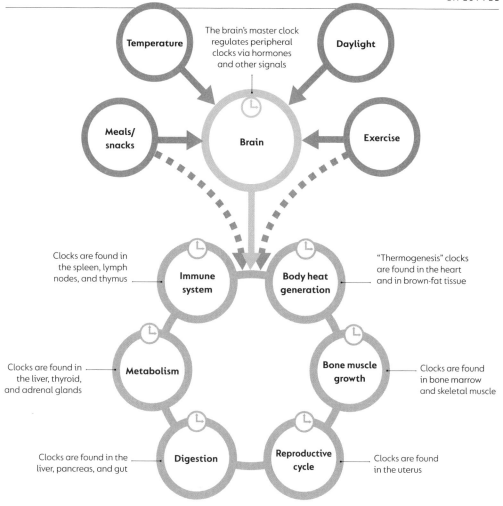

The brain's master clock regulates peripheral clocks via hormones and other signals

Temperature

Daylight

Meals/ snacks

Brain

Exercise

Clocks are found in the spleen, lymph nodes, and thymus

Immune system

Body heat generation

"Thermogenesis" clocks are found in the heart and in brown-fat tissue

Clocks are found in the liver, thyroid, and adrenal glands

Metabolism

Bone muscle growth

Clocks are found in bone marrow and skeletal muscle

Clocks are found in the liver, pancreas, and gut

Digestion

Reproductive cycle

Clocks are found in the uterus

Exercise can also reset your body clock; in a study, people who exercised in the morning or early afternoon were able to advance their body clock and go to sleep earlier. Exercising an hour or two before bed may help delay sleep, too.

Routine is critical to getting your body clocks to run smoothly. Maintain a regular sleep/wake time, get as much natural light as you can in the morning, and keep to consistent times for exercise and meals.

KEY

▬ Zeitgebers
▬ Master clock
▬ Peripheral body clocks

Circadian timing system

This shows the complex relationship between external cues (zeitgebers), the master clock, and the peripheral clocks.

How does shift work affect my sleep?

As we move increasingly to a 24/7 culture, many people now work outside of traditional "office" hours. Night work, extended hours, or rotating between early and late shifts every few days or weeks puts us at odds with our natural circadian rhythms, which are timed to the natural light–dark cycle. For instance, the body produces more of the energizing hormone cortisol in the early morning—this can stop you from falling and staying asleep after a night shift, however physically exhausted you feel.

Some people are genetically more suited to night work, and the body clock may eventually adjust to a regular night shift. But alternating between day and night shifts

Body clock vs. night shift

The body clock releases energizing or sleep-inducing hormones according to the day/night cycle, which means that on night shifts, people work when their bodies are least prepared for physical and mental exertion.

KEY

■ Melatonin level
■ Cortisol level
▧ Alertness level

Melatonin declines and cortisol peaks to prepare for waking

Melatonin is suppressed; mind at peak alertness (9 a.m.–11 a.m.)

Reaction times are fastest (2 p.m.–4 p.m.)

Greatest cardio efficiency and **muscle strength** (5 p.m.)

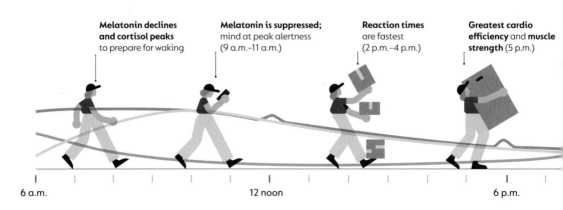

6 a.m.   12 noon   6 p.m.

fights against a regular, healthy sleep schedule; one study showed rotating shift workers get up to four hours less sleep when they sleep during the day.

Short-term circadian disruption results in tiredness, lack of energy, and irritability. For some, it may develop into chronic "shift-work disorder"—feeling excessively sleepy at work yet still being unable to sleep properly at bedtime. This can impair performance; research suggests the risk of accidents in car plants is 30 to 50 percent higher during night shifts. Circadian rhythms also regulate appetite and metabolism, and high-calorie snacking to combat late-night fatigue can lead to weight gain—a study of nurses found that those working rotating shifts were more inclined to be obese.

Longer term, various studies have identified shift work as a contributing factor in health problems such as type 2 diabetes, cardiovascular disease, and strokes. Living out of sync with family and friends may also affect mental well-being, a potential risk factor for depression.

SUPPORT YOUR SCHEDULE

- **Prioritize sleep**, even on days off. If your shifts rotate, toward the end of one phase, go to bed earlier (or later) to prepare your system for the next phase.

- **If you can, work rotating shifts** that move forward in time, as the body tends to prefer a slightly longer cycle to one that is cut short.

- **One or two 20-minute naps** during night shift breaks can improve decision-making and vigilance. A prenap coffee temporarily boosts alertness, too, but avoid caffeine before bed.

- **Eat a balanced meal** before a night shift (but avoid big meals from midnight to 6 a.m., whatever your shift pattern). Preprepare healthy snacks and drink plenty of water.

- **Try moderate exercise** before a night shift to feel more alert. If you're flagging at work, walk or jog around.

- **Wear sunglasses home** after a night shift to delay your brain's switch to daylight mode. Ask your doctor if bright-light therapy (see pages 172–173) could be useful for coping with your schedule.

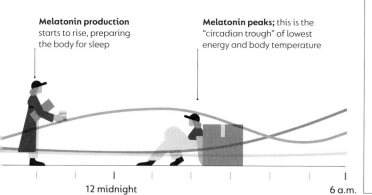

Melatonin production starts to rise, preparing the body for sleep

Melatonin peaks; this is the "circadian trough" of lowest energy and body temperature

12 midnight   6 a.m.

Can I reset my body clock to run earlier or later?

Whether you have to get up earlier for a new job or you want to start exercising first thing for your health, it will take persistence to reset your sleeping pattern. Your biological clock controls when you naturally sleep, wake, and feel most alert in any 24-hour period. The rhythm is influenced by external factors, but it is also programmed by your genes; each of us has a "chronotype" that we can't simply override (see pages 78–79).

Scientists are discovering more about how genes affect our sleep/wake behavior. For example, early bird chronotypes appear to have a longer "PER 3" gene than night owls, which also hardwires early bird types to need more sleep. Most of us are intermediates who lean slightly toward either morning or night.

As you can't beat your biology, it's better to work with your body's natural sleep/wake pattern rather than against it. For instance, will getting up an hour earlier for yoga class suit your chronotype? (See pages 78–79 to find out more.) If the answer is yes because you're naturally an early bird, bear in mind that you will still need to go to bed an hour earlier to ensure your body gets enough restorative sleep.

Routine is critical, too; maintain any new sleep/wake schedule seven days a week. Unless you are an extreme chronotype, your body should gradually adapt to the new timetable as long as you consistently get enough rest.

MAKING THE SHIFT

• **Introduce changes gradually**. See opposite for a four-week plan to bring your body clock forward or back by an hour.

• **To help your system fire up** earlier, go outside into the daylight as soon as possible after you get up. And to

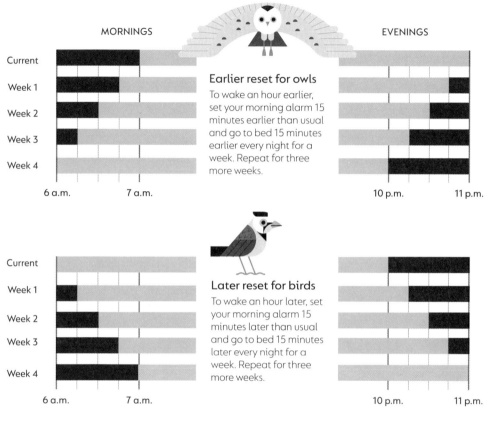

MORNINGS

EVENINGS

Earlier reset for owls

To wake an hour earlier, set your morning alarm 15 minutes earlier than usual and go to bed 15 minutes earlier every night for a week. Repeat for three more weeks.

Current
Week 1
Week 2
Week 3
Week 4

6 a.m.   7 a.m.

10 p.m.   11 p.m.

Later reset for birds

To wake an hour later, set your morning alarm 15 minutes later than usual and go to bed 15 minutes later every night for a week. Repeat for three more weeks.

Current
Week 1
Week 2
Week 3
Week 4

6 a.m.   7 a.m.

10 p.m.   11 p.m.

reinforce an earlier body clock reset, try eating something right after you wake up. You may not feel like it at first, but do it every day and your biological clock will in time change its circadian pattern so that hunger will help wake you at the new earlier time.

- **It isn't possible to make major changes** in your hard-wired clock—an hour either way is the most you can realistically aim for. A major lifestyle change, like permanent night shift work, will be more challenging. (For more on managing shifts and night work, see pages 146–147.)

KEY

▨ Waking time
■ Sleeping time

Why do I feel groggy when I've had more sleep than usual?

You've treated yourself to sleeping in, only to wake up feeling fuzzy-headed and lethargic. Infuriatingly, all that extra sleep has left you drained instead of refreshed.

Changes in your sleep routine confuse the body's internal clock, which coordinates the chemical, hormonal, and temperature changes that power up your system before you wake. If you wake later than normal, you miss the energizing effects of the hormone cortisol, which peaks in the early morning. Also, by sleeping later, you enter a new cycle of sleep, and if you wake during the deepest phase of this cycle, you'll feel extremely groggy—a condition known as sleep inertia. This can last from a few minutes to three hours, and evidence suggests that its effects can feel like the equivalent of 40 hours of sleep deprivation.

AVOID HITTING "SNOOZE"

You may have noticed sleep inertia when you hit snooze on your alarm and drop off again. Snoozing gives the brain time to enter a new sleep phase, and if you're then jerked awake from deep sleep, the brain takes far longer to enter the conscious world. Be mindful of this if you're planning to nap before driving or doing a challenging task, because you won't react as fast or think quite as clearly as normal. Research suggests sleep inertia is most likely if you nap for longer than 30 minutes, but it may be less if you're already sleep-deprived.

For most people, a regular sleep routine will prevent sleep inertia becoming a problem. Severe morning sleep inertia (also known as "sleep drunkenness") can also involve confusion and even aggression.

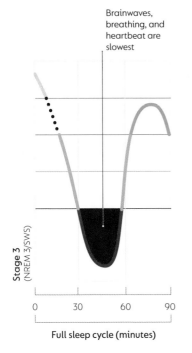

Brainwaves, breathing, and heartbeat are slowest

Stage 3
(NREM 3/SWS)

0   30   60   90

Full sleep cycle (minutes)

Danger zone
Jolting awake from the deepest sleep stage puts stress on the body and disorients the brain.

Does altitude help or hinder sleep?

Because most of us aren't used to living at high altitudes, arriving at these destinations can disrupt the body's systems and lead to problems with sleep.

There's not a lot of research around how altitude impacts sleep, but the reduced level of oxygen at high altitudes means that breathing often becomes difficult. The nausea, headaches, and dizziness this brings are symptoms of what is known as altitude sickness. It's thought this oxygen deprivation also causes significant sleep fragmentation and a reduction in deeper, slow-wave restorative sleep.

When oxygen in the blood falls below a certain level as you sleep, the body experiences hypoxia: it starts to work harder to take in more oxygen and expel carbon dioxide by alternating between rapid and slow breathing. It's when your breathing slows or even stops briefly that you wake up. These constant interruptions stop you from reaching the deeper stages of sleep needed to feel fully rested.

SLEEP WELL AT ALTITUDE

Specific treatments for sleep disorders at altitude are scarce, but the steps that help prevent altitude sickness can also improve sleep quality after a few days. Extra oxygen and taking a nitrate supplement, such as beet juice, may help. Some doctors prescribe acetazolamide and nonbenzodiazepine medications that reduce periodic breathing, which in turn helps improve sleep quality.

It's essential at high altitudes to drink plenty of water during the day, eat a diet that's high in carbohydrates (the most easily accessed form of energy for your body), and avoid tobacco and alcohol, both of which can make breathing more difficult.

Before traveling, ask your doctor for advice and look up local remedies for altitude sickness at your destination.

Height above sea level (feet)

- 20,000
- Domar, China 16,142 ft (4,920 m)
- La Paz, Bolivia 12,694 ft (3,869 m)
- Cusco, Peru 11,152 ft (3,399 m)
- 10,000
- Quito, Ecuador 9,350 ft (2,850 m)
- Mexico City, Mexico 7,382 ft (2,250 m)
- 5,200
- Kathmandu, Nepal 4,593 ft (1,400 m)
- Jerusalem, Israel 2,474 ft (754 m)
- Paris, France 115 ft (35 m)
- 0

KEY
- Altitude sickness zone
- Altitude range of 95% of settlements

Sleeping at high elevation
Those who live more than 10,000 ft (3,000 m) above sea level are used to sleeping in their high-altitude homes. However, the vast majority of people live less than 5,200 ft (1,600 m) above sea level, and visiting high regions can affect sleep.

Are there foods and drinks that help you sleep?

One of the most widely held beliefs about sleep is that a glass of milk just before bed will send you off into a peaceful slumber—but what does the science say? When it comes to food or drink and sleeping, there are two factors at play: what you consume and how and when you consume it. (See pages 86–87 and 162–163 for more on eating behaviors and sleep patterns.)

There are compounds found in certain foods and drinks that may help us either fall or stay asleep. One of these is tryptophan, an amino acid that the brain converts into serotonin, the feel-good hormone, which is in turn converted to melatonin, the sleep-inducing hormone. Our body doesn't make tryptophan, so we have to get it from our diet. One of the main sources of tryptophan is indeed milk, so that old wives' tale is true.

Some foods are also rich in melatonin or contain minerals, such as magnesium, that prepare the brain for sleep. Some high-fiber foods have also been found to decrease the time it takes us to fall asleep and increase the amount of time spent in deeper, slow-wave, restorative sleep—possibly because they prevent blood sugar surges, which can lower melatonin levels.

There are also key food culprits that will keep you awake or impair sleep quality. Caffeine (see pages 154–155), for example, interferes with the urge to sleep, while food or drink that triggers digestive upsets or increases your need for the bathroom in the night will prevent continuous sleep (see pages 140–141).

Research into the sleep-inducing properties of food is a complex and ongoing process, but based on what we know so far, upping your intake of fruits, vegetables, whole grains, nuts, and lean proteins should help you experience longer, better-quality sleep.

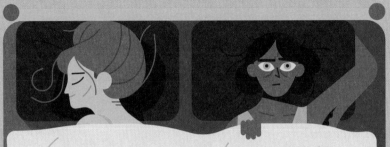

Help or hinder?

Food and drink can play a role in both the quantity and quality of our sleep, so choose what you consume wisely!

Helps you sleep

Tryptophan
Found in: milk, oats, cashew nuts, lean chicken, turkey, and lamb

Melatonin
Found in: eggs, fish, nuts, brown mushrooms, cereals, and seeds

Magnesium
Found in: green leafy veggies, nuts, and whole grains

Fiber
Found in: whole grains, oats, asparagus, and broccoli

Keeps you awake

Caffeine
Blocks the brain's natural sleep drive, especially if consumed too close to bedtime

Alcohol
Impairs REM sleep, which is important for memory and learning

Spicy foods
Contain capsaicin and may increase body temperature, which can interfere with sleep

Sugary or fatty foods
High-sugar foods and unsaturated fats reduce time in deep, restorative sleep

153

Is caffeine really sleep's no. 1 enemy?

Caffeine is one of the most widely used drugs in the world. For some people, it's a kick-start to the day, whereas others report it does nothing for them. So how exactly does caffeine impact sleep?

Caffeine shows up everywhere, not only in food and drink, but also in toiletries, medications, and even in cosmetics. It can improve our performance, consolidate memory, and wake us up when we feel drowsy—and it's this last fact that causes problems when it comes to sleep.

CAFFEINE AND THE BRAIN

Caffeine is a stimulant, triggering the release of adrenaline, the fight-or-flight hormone, which is why you experience a burst of energy when it enters your system. It also interferes with how the brain responds to the chemical adenosine. An essential piece in the sleep-wake puzzle, adenosine slows the central nervous system, building the urge to sleep (see pages 24–25) as night approaches. Caffeine binds to the same brain receptors as adenosine, blocking the signals that make us feel sleepy. Everyone's adenosine receptors differ due to genetics—so if caffeine doesn't affect you, it may be you don't have very "sticky" receptors for caffeine to bind to.

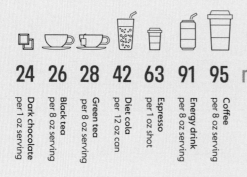

24	26	28	42	63	91	95	mg
Dark chocolate per 1 oz serving	Black tea per 8 oz serving	Green tea per 8 oz serving	Diet cola per 12 oz can	Espresso per 1 oz shot	Energy drink per 8 oz serving	Coffee per 8 oz serving	

Caffeine league table

There can be a surprisingly high level of caffeine in everyday drinks and food. Based on average servings, coffee and energy drinks score highest, but there's plenty lurking in cola, tea (including "healthy" green tea), and dark chocolate.

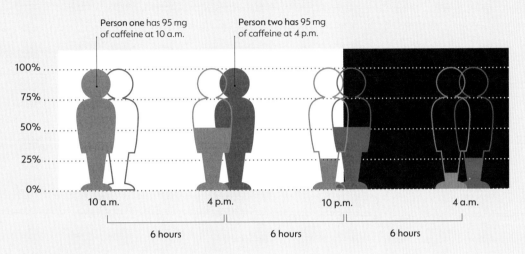

Person one has 95 mg of caffeine at 10 a.m.

Person two has 95 mg of caffeine at 4 p.m.

100%
75%
50%
25%
0%

| 10 a.m. | 4 p.m. | 10 p.m. | 4 a.m. |

6 hours   6 hours   6 hours

Rate of decline

Having caffeine earlier in the day gives your body a better chance of clearing it from adenosine receptors before sleep. Drinking coffee at 10 a.m. rather than 4 p.m. means less will remain in your system by 10 p.m.

THE HALF-LIFE OF CAFFEINE

The level of caffeine in your body drops by 50 percent roughly every six hours, so half of the caffeine from a 4 p.m. cup of coffee will still be circulating in your system at 10 p.m., blocking adenosine and making it a prime suspect as the cause of poor sleep. It's not easy to gauge just how much caffeine you are consuming, so make sure you check the levels in your food and drink, especially if you know you are sensitive to its effects. Stick to a daily limit of 300 mg of caffeine (around three cups of coffee) for adults and less than 85 mg (one soft drink and one cup of tea) for children. You should also try to have your last caffeine fix by mid-afternoon so that most of it has been cleared from your system before you go to bed.

CAFFEINE-FREE ENERGY BOOSTS

• **Step out for 10 minutes** A brisk walk will clear your head and reboot your system naturally. The added benefit is that you get a bit more exercise into your day, which will also help you sleep better at night.

• **Drink more water** Water can boost concentration by helping flush the brain of toxins. It also oxygenates brain cells, improving alertness.

Can multivitamins help me sleep?

The question of how and to what extent vitamins interact with the biological processes involved in sleep is subject to ongoing research.

Vitamins are the essential nutrients found in food that play an important role in many of our bodily functions. So far, there's no evidence that taking a combined multivitamin supplement will promote sleep, but it may be that certain individual vitamins can play a positive role.

SLEEP-FRIENDLY VITAMINS

Vitamin D is naturally produced by the skin in response to sunlight, and studies show that people with lower levels of vitamin D seem to have poorer sleep—although why this is the case is not yet fully understood. What we do know is that sunlight is a key regulator of our circadian rhythms, so spending just 10 minutes outside each day will boost vitamin D levels and also support your natural body clock.

Vitamin B6 seems to be important for the hormones we need for sleep, triggering serotonin production, which is then converted to melatonin, the sleepiness hormone.

Interestingly, the role vitamins play in good sleep may actually be down to how they address underlying issues that cause poor sleep. Both vitamin C and D seem to relieve sleep apnea, possibly because they boost circulation and decrease inflammation; and, as vitamin B6 plays a role in mood, it can be useful for those with depression, which is a major cause of poor sleep. In some cases, too much of a vitamin can be an issue; an excess of vitamin B12 has been linked to insomnia.

The simplest way to get all the vitamins you need is to eat a well-balanced diet, but certain vitamins can be useful to address some specific sleep issues. Always consult your doctor before taking any supplements.

" "

In winter, when there's less sunlight, taking extra vitamin D may improve your sleep.

156

Does alcohol help or harm my sleep?

Alcohol is a sedative—it slows brain function and induces drowsiness. However, it's not recommended as a sleeping aid, as it disrupts natural sleep cycles. When alcohol enters your system, it triggers a release of endorphins (feel-good hormones) in the parts of the brain associated with pleasure and reward. Once this passes, alcohol soon becomes a sedative, so you might think this would result in a good night's sleep—but actually the opposite is true. As the body processes alcohol, you reach deeper, slow-wave Stage-3 sleep more quickly, but this comes at the expense of REM, the most restorative stage of slumber. In the middle of the night, once the alcohol has been processed, you experience "REM rebound," where REM increases in a bid to catch up and maintain your normal sleep patterns, but this usually disrupts your natural waking process.

Alcohol is also a diuretic, so you're more likely to need to get up to urinate during the night. High consumption can also trigger snoring, sleep apnea, and sleepwalking, all of which further disrupt sleep.

The effects of alcohol

An alcohol-affected sleep pattern looks markedly different from a typical night's sleep. You can see that alcohol creates an imbalance between Stage-3 and REM sleep, which results in a disrupted, poor-quality night's rest.

KEY

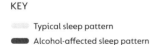

Typical sleep pattern
Alcohol-affected sleep pattern

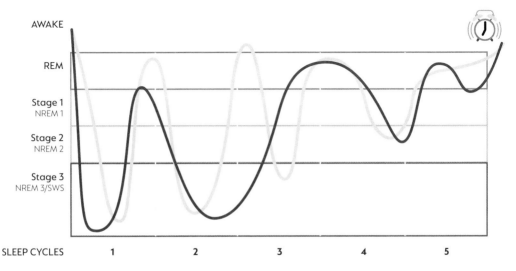

| | AWAKE |
| REM |
| Stage 1 NREM 1 |
| Stage 2 NREM 2 |
| Stage 3 NREM 3/SWS |

SLEEP CYCLES   1   2   3   4   5

Do CBD products help with sleep?

In the last few years, there's been a surge in cannabidiol (CBD) products that claim to cure insomnia—but evidence to support these claims is thin.

CBD is a chemical compound extracted from the cannabis plant, but CBD has no psychoactive effects—you don't feel intoxicated if you take it. CBD acts on the pleasure receptors in the brain known as the endocannabinoid system, and some research has found it encourages relaxation while lessening anxiety and pain. It's important to note that the legal position of CBD is complex worldwide; some countries ban or limit its use altogether, so you need to know its status where you live or in any country you are traveling to.

SCAM OR SOLUTION?

Despite the reported benefits, there's limited evidence to support the use of CBD products for sleep problems, and current research indicates that, while CBD may lessen some of the indirect causes of poor sleep (such as stress), it has no beneficial effect on the mechanics of sleep. It's not yet clear whether the benefits that some users report are genuine or a result of the "placebo effect."

It can also be difficult to be sure what's really in many of the products claiming to contain CBD. In most countries, its manufacture is unregulated, which makes it difficult to ensure products are safe or doses are consistent.

Weighing up all these factors, it's not recommended to take CBD for sleep problems. Getting to the crux of why you are not sleeping rather than masking any symptoms you may have is really the only surefire way to combat sleeplessness in the long term.

How does smoking affect my sleep?

When it comes to sleep, it's the nicotine in smoking products that poses the main problem for smokers. Nicotine is an addictive stimulant, produced by the nightshade family of plants, that increases alertness. Studies show that nicotine use results in difficulties falling and staying asleep, and also decreases overall sleep quality—smokers experience more broken sleep and less slow-wave, restorative sleep than nonsmokers.

Some smokers also report that they are awakened by nighttime nicotine cravings. The nicotine they take in then keeps them from falling asleep again, setting up a cycle of sleeplessness. This is why smoking is often a significant risk factor in developing insomnia—chronic sleeplessness.

Smoking also increases your chances of suffering from sleep apnea, where breathing is constantly disrupted during the night, making you wake repeatedly. This is because smoke irritates tissues in the nose and throat, causing swelling that can impede your airway.

WHAT ABOUT VAPING?

Most vapers use products containing nicotine—and the nicotine "hit" can be more potent than from a cigarette. If you are vaping to help you quit smoking, consider switching to an e-liquid with a lower nicotine strength during the day and a nicotine-free type in the evening. This will give your body a window to clear stimulating nicotine from your system before you are ready to sleep.

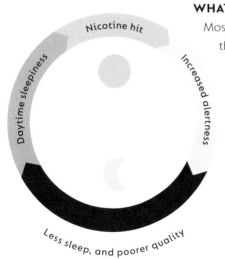

A cycle of poor sleep

The effects of nicotine both disrupt and curtail sleep, which results in excessive daytime sleepiness. People then smoke to boost their alertness, and this in turn prevents and disrupts sleep the following night.

Is a bath before bed helpful for relaxation and sleep?

Taking a bath can be a great way to relax, and there's clinical evidence to suggest that—depending on temperature and timing—it can greatly benefit sleep. A warm bath can help you fall asleep quicker, as once you get out of the bathtub, your body temperature drops rapidly, triggering the release of the sleepiness hormone melatonin. However, if the bath is too hot, this could actually inhibit melatonin production; keep water at a temperature that is pleasant but doesn't make you sweat.

You don't have to soak for hours to get the benefit—research indicates that just 10 minutes in a warm bath before bed can increase slow-wave sleep and sleep duration. Warm water also helps activate the parasympathetic nervous system (PNS), our built-in stress-relief response, reducing levels of cortisol, a drop that is essential for sleep onset. Warm water additionally relaxes muscles and relieves tension and joint pain—all of which set you up for a good night's rest.

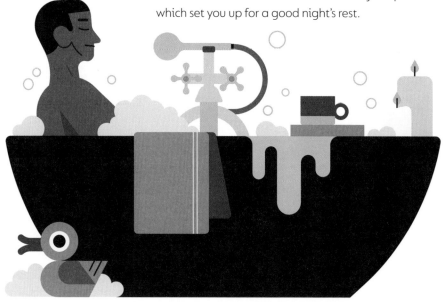

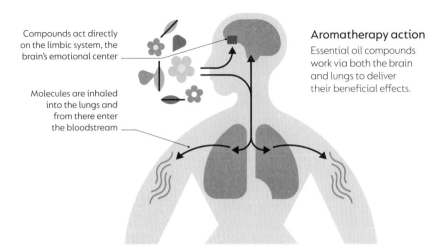

Compounds act directly on the limbic system, the brain's emotional center

Molecules are inhaled into the lungs and from there enter the bloodstream

Aromatherapy action
Essential oil compounds work via both the brain and lungs to deliver their beneficial effects.

Do essential oils help with sleep?

The aromatic extracts of plants have long been used to encourage rest and relaxation, and research has confirmed that some essential oils do in fact aid sleep. Certain essential oils have been recorded as having a particularly beneficial effect on sleep. For example, in one hospital study, patients who had aromatherapy treatments with lavender essential oil experienced less daytime drowsiness and enjoyed more consistent sleep at night—possibly because the compounds found in lavender have a proven sedative effect on the nervous system.

Essential oils can be administered in a variety of ways: into the air via a diffuser or room spray, inhaled directly via a handy "aromastick" or a tissue sprinkled with oil, or diluted in a neutral carrier oil and used as a massage or bath oil.

Never put undiluted essential oil directly on the skin, and if you are pregnant or have any underlying health conditions, always seek the advice of a qualified practitioner before use.

SLEEP-INDUCING OILS

Many essential oils contain compounds that studies have found to have a calming effect on the body's stress response. These include bergamot, ylang-ylang, chamomile, lavender, and frankincense.

Will late-evening eating affect my sleep?

If you want to fall asleep easily and enjoy a good night's rest, there are a few reasons why going to bed with a full stomach isn't the best strategy.

For some, a snack before bedtime wards off any midnight hunger pangs, but for many, late-night eating triggers digestive problems such as heartburn. The key is to be mindful of what you eat to ensure you are comfortable before you head to bed—getting horizontal too soon after a meal, especially if that meal has been large, spicy, or fatty, could keep you from getting to sleep.

Support circadian health

Taking your meals within an 8–12-hour window can support your natural digestive body clock, which in turn helps you get restful sleep. There is evidence that restricted eating windows can help maintain metabolic health, too.

THE DIGESTIVE BODY CLOCK

It's not only sleeping and waking that are controlled by your internal rhythms; the digestive system is also regulated by your 24-hour clock. Eating a meal close to bedtime can mean you fire up your digestion just when the body is preparing to put its systems into "rest mode" for the night. One way to help your digestive and sleep body clocks stay synchronized is to keep to a meal schedule that allows your digestive system to rest when you do. There is evidence to suggest that a time-restricted pattern of eating can be beneficial in helping you achieve this; eating regularly within a similar window of time each day allows your body to process food when its digestive functions are at their peak, so it can spend the rest of the time recovering. We all have different metabolisms, schedules, and lifestyles, so figure out what works best for you to ensure you have processed your food before you sleep. If you need to eat later, then keep your meal or snack light so it is fully digested before bed.

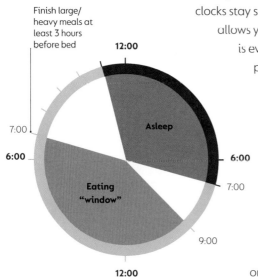

Finish large/ heavy meals at least 3 hours before bed

12:00

Asleep

7:00

6:00

6:00

7:00

Eating "window"

9:00

12:00

" "   _____

One study found that
participants who ate a
meal close to bedtime
took longer to fall asleep
than those who ate
earlier in the evening.

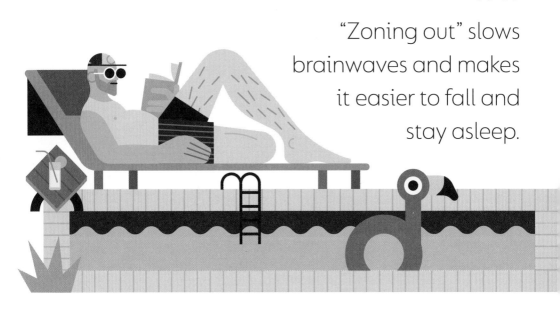

" "
"Zoning out" slows brainwaves and makes it easier to fall and stay asleep.

Why do I sleep better on vacation?

For many of us, a vacation is one of the few opportunities we get to completely relax. Many of us feel we sleep better when we go away, and science backs this up.

Picture your ideal vacation: your days are stress-free, you fall asleep minutes after your head hits the pillow, and you wake the next morning feeling refreshed. If your sleep improves on vacation, it's likely because, for once, you are physically and mentally in the right state for good sleep.

EXPOSURE TO DAYLIGHT

Morning light is essential to regulate the sleep/wake cycle and to build sleep pressure (see page 108). On vacation, we often get more exposure to light in the morning, maybe because we are in a destination with longer daylight hours or simply because we seize the day and get out earlier. This keeps our circadian rhythms on track and makes it more likely we will get good sleep at night.

CAREFREE AND RELAXED

Away from the constraints and obligations of daily life, people's stress levels usually decrease, enabling sleep-influencing hormones to work optimally. Also, freeing yourself from the need to be "busy" can encourage deep mental relaxation, or "zoning out." This mildly hypnotic state has proven beneficial effects on both brain and body, enhancing your chances of good sleep.

Being on vacation can also mean you are more sociable than usual, taking time to enjoy the company of others. Positive social interaction can raise levels of oxytocin (the "love hormone"), leaving you feeling good, as well as further reducing the cortisol circulating in your body. One recent study that measured people's sleep after eating out with friends found that their quality of sleep significantly improved following this social contact.

Finally, a vacation is a change of scenery, and this break from any negative sleep associations and habits you might have formed at home can offer you a chance to mentally wipe the slate clean and sleep well.

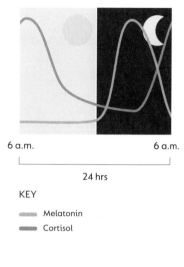

6 a.m.   6 a.m.

24 hrs

KEY

Melatonin

Cortisol

Vacation hormones

In a low-stress environment, cortisol stays low during the day and evening, enabling a healthy surge of sleepiness-inducing melatonin as night approaches.

TAKE VACATION SLEEP HOME

If you want to sleep better when you're home from your travels, try to find ways to add those vacation habits to your routine.

• **Make time for slowing down** Although it's tempting to cram your daily schedule, try to fight the urge and give yourself permission to do less—keeping mind and body as calm and stress-free as possible is crucial to good sleep.

• **Get outdoors** Being outside more during the day—and especially in the morning—means more exposure to daylight, which helps regulate natural sleep rhythms.

• **Switch off** Make time to wind down in the evenings by doing something sociable or relaxing in the few hours before you head to bed. This will help your body ensure its balance of hormones is optimal for sleep.

How can I manage my sleep across time zones?

"Jet lag" is a disruption to your body clock that is triggered by traveling to a different time zone. This shift can interfere significantly with sleep. When your internal clock doesn't line up with the time at your destination, this can lead to trouble. Depending on the time zone, you might find it difficult to get to sleep, or you may be overwhelmingly sleepy in the middle of the day and find you're wide awake at 3 a.m.

You may suffer jet lag if you travel across two or more time zones—the more you cross, the more disruption to your body clock—but there are steps you can take to minimize the effects. If possible in the week or so before traveling, start to readjust your body clock by gradually moving your times for eating and sleeping nearer to those at your destination.

Time traveling

The direction in which you are traveling and how far are the two key factors determining how jet lag might affect your sleep at your destination.

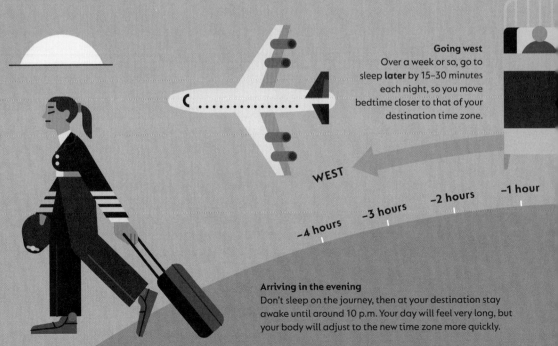

Going west
Over a week or so, go to sleep **later** by 15–30 minutes each night, so you move bedtime closer to that of your destination time zone.

WEST

−4 hours   −3 hours   −2 hours   −1 hour

Arriving in the evening
Don't sleep on the journey, then at your destination stay awake until around 10 p.m. Your day will feel very long, but your body will adjust to the new time zone more quickly.

Just before the flight, change your watch to the time at your destination to further readjust your body clock. Research has also shown that fasting just before and during travel can help reset your clock, likely because eating is a key zeitgeber—an event that cues the timing of circadian rhythms such as sleeping and waking.

Jet lag is usually worse when traveling east: time zones are ahead of your body clock, so at bedtime you are wide awake. It takes longer for the body clock to reset. Traveling west, time zones are behind your body clock, so bedtime is later than your body expects. This is usually easier to adjust to than a too-early bedtime. Getting plenty of daylight at your destination and sleeping at an appropriate time for the new time zone will help your body clock adapt.

APPS OR SUPPLEMENTS?

Apps can help you manage jet lag by analyzing your personal sleep pattern, chronotype, and travel itinerary, then creating a tailor-made schedule for you based on the data. There is some evidence that taking a melatonin supplement may help shift the body clock; see page 101 for more on melatonin and how to use it.

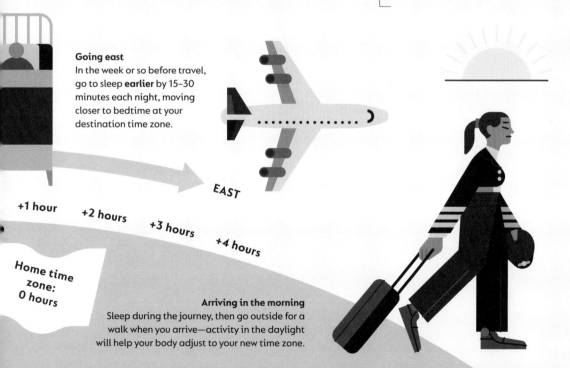

Going east
In the week or so before travel, go to sleep **earlier** by 15–30 minutes each night, moving closer to bedtime at your destination time zone.

EAST

+1 hour   +2 hours   +3 hours   +4 hours

Home time zone:
0 hours

Arriving in the morning
Sleep during the journey, then go outside for a walk when you arrive—activity in the daylight will help your body adjust to your new time zone.

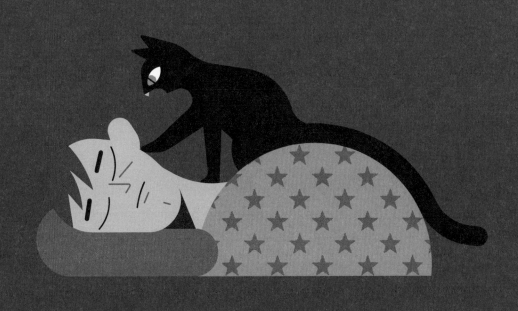

Your sleep environment

Sleep is a sensory process, and factors such as light, noise, bedding, and temperature can all influence your sleep experience. For many of us, there is much we can do to our external sleep environment to make drifting off easier and to ensure our sleep is uninterrupted.

Declutter your space

A tidy, clear space will help you empty your mind. It's hard to relax if you are constantly reminded of unfinished chores.

Choose the right bedding

You need to be cool enough to fall asleep, then warm enough to stay asleep. Bed linens in breathable fibers will help regulate your temperature.

Create a scent-sation

Lavender essential oil, used either in a room diffuser or mixed with water and sprayed on a pillow, is proven to increase slow-wave restorative sleep.

Keep the lights low

As evening wears on, dim the lights to aid your natural sleepiness.

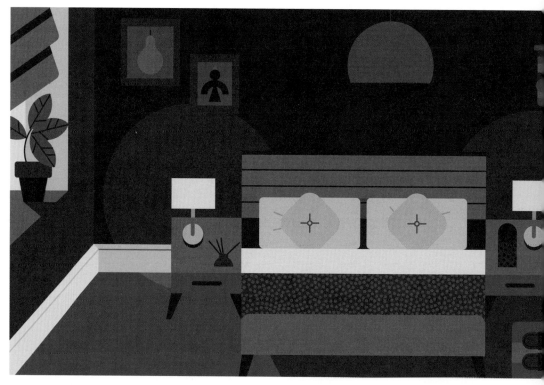

Listen and sleep

While looking at screens can overstimulate you, listening to a soothing story, podcast, or nature sounds can induce calm and aid sleep.

Green your bedroom

Houseplants can purify the air. The calathea closes its leaves at night and opens in the morning, reflecting our own body rhythms.

Wake with the day

If waking up feels like a chore, leave the curtains open to allow the morning light to boost your waking hormones.

Make the bed

Making your bed as soon as you rise helps you mentally shake off the night; your bed will also look more inviting for the next sleep.

How do I make my bedroom a sleep sanctuary?

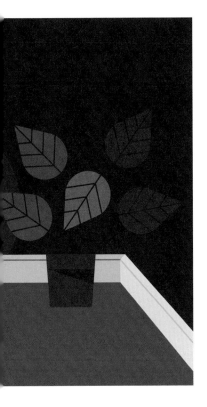

Your bedroom should be a refuge from the demands of daily life, a serene space to begin your day in, and a haven to retreat to at night to rest and recharge. When thinking about making your bedroom a sleep sanctuary, approach it as a sensory process, ensuring that all your senses are soothed and satisfied by the environment you create. This in turn will dial down your stress—by avoiding overstimulation via your senses, you ensure body and mind are primed for rest.

CREATING A SENSORY OASIS

• **Sight** Is your room a pleasure to look at? Do you look at your bed and want to dive in? If not, it's time to make changes—and it doesn't have to be costly to make your room a sight for sore eyes.

• **Touch** Whatever comes into contact with your skin should feel good—be it bed linens, pillows, nightwear, or the carpet under your feet. Your skin is the largest organ in your body and a major indicator of your comfort level.

• **Sound** Your bedroom's soundscape will play a big part in your prospects of good rest. Street sounds can jerk you into consciousness and may be a stress trigger, but for others, complete silence is unnerving and maintains wakefulness. Figure out what works best for you.

• **Smell** Scent signals from the olfactory nerves connect directly to the brain's emotional center, so they can have an impact on sleep. Make sure your bedroom smells inviting—dirty sports clothes in the bottom of the laundry basket or the lingering odor of a late-night snack is unlikely to promote restorative sleep.

Why do I need more sleep in the winter?

When nights draw in and days shorten, many people feel sluggish and want to stay curled up in bed in the morning. There's a reason you may feel you need more sleep in winter. Humans are programmed to respond to light and other external cues—called zeitgebers—that influence our internal body clock. In winter, we live with shorter days and less bright sunlight, which can throw off the timing of our normal sleep/wake cycle, affecting our energy levels.

Some of us find it particularly hard to adjust to seasonal changes, especially going into fall and winter. As many as one in five people experience one or more symptoms of "seasonal affective disorder" (SAD), which is a type of recurring depression. While mild cases are often called "winter blues," some sufferers are so badly affected that they can't function properly during winter months.

Scientists aren't certain what causes SAD, but one theory is that sufferers' circadian rhythms react more slowly to light cues, so they are less able to regulate their bodies' melatonin and serotonin, which affect sleep and mood. A study found 80 percent of SAD patients suffered from "hypersomnia," or regular oversleeping with daytime drowsiness and napping; more than half reported sleeping

The gray regions on this map, north and south of the tropics, are most affected by SAD

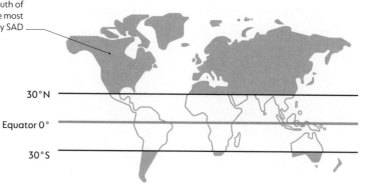

Winter daylight hours

In winter, the days are short and the nights long at latitudes more than 30° north or south of the equator, with the poles seeing almost no daylight. Limited daylight can lead to SAD, and consequently poor sleep.

30°N

Equator 0°

30°S

more than two hours extra per night in winter. Research in Finland suggests people with winter-onset SAD are at a greater risk of frequent nightmares and insomnia. Other symptoms of winter SAD include increased appetite and a craving for carbohydrates, lethargy and low activity levels, inability to concentrate, sadness, and frequent crying.

WINTER COPING STRATEGIES

• **Make the most of natural sunlight.** Take daily 10-minute walks outside and, when indoors, sit by a window if you can.

• **Try to stick to the same sleep/wake routine** and sleep for the same amount of time as you would in summer.

• **Exercise** is known to help improve mood, and timing it regularly will help get your circadian rhythm on track.

• **Bright-light therapy** is a proven treatment for SAD. In the morning, users sit near a lightbox that produces very bright light to mimic sunlight. This stimulates the brain's neurotransmitters and helps restore normal circadian rhythm. Always use light therapy under the guidance of a doctor or sleep professional.

SUMMER "WHITE NIGHTS"

The 24-hour daylight of high-latitude summers brings its own sleep challenges. In Norway, Oslo gets 19 hours' peak summer sunshine, while north of the Arctic Circle the sun doesn't set on Tromsø from May to July. Without the cue of fading daylight to activate the sleepiness hormone melatonin, many people find getting to sleep during light nights a real problem. Wearing sunglasses in the evening to block out light has been found to help improve sleep.

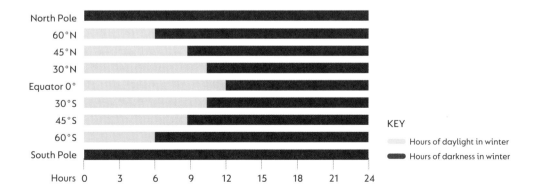

KEY

▭ Hours of daylight in winter
▬ Hours of darkness in winter

Can the full moon affect my sleep?

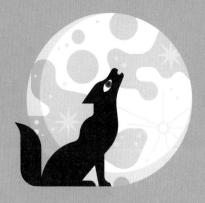

For centuries, the full moon has been a focus of fascination and superstition—including the idea that it can play havoc with our sleep.

All kinds of phenomena have been blamed on the full moon, from mythical werewolves to increased crime, sleep problems, and even insanity—the term "lunatic" derives from the Latin *lunaticus*, meaning "moonstruck."

It's true that when it comes to nature, lunar rhythms certainly do have an effect; the difference between high and low ocean tides is greatest during a full moon as the earth's gravitational pull increases, and the annual mass spawning of coral on Australia's Great Barrier Reef follows a full moon each winter. However, when it comes to humans, there's limited scientific evidence that a full moon affects our behavior in quite the way legend would have us believe.

The association between a full moon and poor sleep might not be down to anything mysterious or supernatural, but something much simpler—an example of what's known as confirmation bias. This is when you are more likely to engage with and remember information that fits with your existing beliefs. So if you slept badly and noticed it was a full moon, rather than thinking it a coincidence, you take it as confirmation of the moon's eerie powers—conveniently forgetting any sleeplessness you've had on nights on which there was not a full moon.

The moon is also a source of light, and as light can trigger our wake response (see pages 172–173), it's maybe unsurprising that in communities without artificial light at night, a full moon can have a sleep-interrupting effect. Given this, if you live in a city, it's unlikely a full moon will impact your sleep, but if you're in a more rural, darker area, then draw your curtains well to ensure it doesn't!

Does blue light affect sleep?

Any kind of light can potentially interfere with your ability to fall asleep, but is blue light of the type digital devices emit particularly problematic for sleep?

Light plays a key role in sleeping and waking. Our eyes track the rise and fall of the sun, sending signals to the brain to tell it to produce various hormones at different times of the day to regulate our sleep/wake cycle (see pages 172–173).

There's some evidence to suggest that due to its short wavelength, blue light is more readily absorbed by the receptors in our eyes—making us more sensitive to its effects than we are to lights of other hues.

CONFUSING YOUR INTERNAL CLOCK?

From this, a theory has gained ground that exposure to blue light from digital devices at night can therefore trick the brain into thinking it's daytime—preventing production of the sleep hormone melatonin and disrupting natural sleepiness. While this is hypothetically possible, in reality, the amount of light digital screens give off is minimal and likely not bright enough to fool our body clock. Blue light is simply no match for natural light when it comes to controlling our sleep rhythms, so a glance at your smartphone in the middle of the night won't have your body believing it's already morning.

Most people are exposed to enough natural light each day to offset any effects digital blue light may have, but if you don't get a lot of natural daylight (for example, if you work night shifts), then you may already struggle with regulating your sleep/wake cycle. In this case, blue light could delay sleep onset for you, so try reducing your digital device usage a couple of hours before bedtime.

SHOULD I USE BLUE-LIGHT FILTERS?

Although blue light is unlikely to interfere with your sleep, there is evidence that it causes extra strain on the eyes. If you spend a lot of time on screens, using blue-light-filtering glasses or screen protectors that block and absorb some of this light could help prevent eye discomfort.

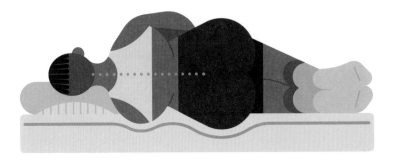

Best for backs
A position in which neck, chest, and lower back are in line keeps the spine aligned and relaxed, minimizing back pain.

What kind of mattress and pillow is best?

We spend one-third of our lives sleeping, so it's worth spending time selecting the right mattress and pillows. Before choosing a new mattress, notice how you feel on waking up. Is your shoulder or lower back aching? Are you too warm? What position are you in? Whether you're a side, back, or stomach sleeper, the ideal mattress will support and align the spine and neck and be comfortable enough to minimize pressure on hips, shoulders, or other contact points.

Mattress fillings include memory foam, springs, gels, and latex, plus hybrid multilayer mattresses, all varying from soft to extra-firm support. "Orthopedic" versions offer firmer support and spread weight evenly, while memory foam molds to the body's curves to relieve pressure but may allow the spine to drop. Hybrids can provide a good support–comfort balance. Foam and latex trap body heat, unlike wool or gel; these can promote better sleep, for instance, during menopause. Hybrids, pocket (individually wrapped) springs, foam, and mattresses incorporating different support levels can reduce motion disturbance from your partner moving on the other side of the bed.

For pillows, back sleepers should choose a type that won't push their head too far forward; front and side sleepers need a firm pillow that helps keep the neck and spine aligned.

Can weighted blankets help with sleep?

Weighted blankets, which contain beads or pellets, are claimed to promote relaxation and calm. They tap into the concept of feel-good pressure by applying weight onto the skin to simulate the feeling of a hug. The theory is that the blanket creates this effect via "proprioceptive deep pressure stimulation." The skin, muscles, and joints have receptors that respond to heat, cold, pain, and pressure—proprioception is the term for the process by which they respond and message the brain, giving the body a physical awareness of itself.

Under pressure

To the body's skin sensors, there is little difference between pressure from a blanket and that of human touch—the brain receives the same signals.

Weight presses onto the skin

"Pacinian corpuscles" sense pressure changes

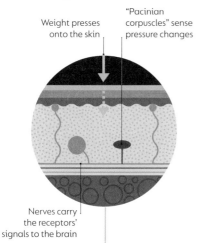

Nerves carry the receptors' signals to the brain

WILL IT HELP ME SLEEP?

It is believed that the pressure of a weighted blanket sitting on the body activates the parasympathetic (or stress-reducing) nervous system, triggering the brain to release neurotransmitters, including serotonin and dopamine. These have a calming effect, reducing anxiety, heart rate, and cortisol, which helps promote sleep.

Research into these blankets' effect on sleep is limited, but a study showed they did improve insomnia in patients with specific psychiatric conditions. While a weighted blanket may improve some sleep problems, if you have sleep apnea or a respiratory condition, the extra weight could further restrict your lungs' ability to expand. If you want to try one, it's a good idea to consult your doctor first.

177

Does the position of my bed affect how well I sleep?

Environmental factors such as light, noise, and temperature all have an impact on our sleep quality—but what about the position of the bed?

There's little research exploring the preferences of bed positions in humans, but it's a fact that we share the same survival instincts as animals in preferring to sleep in a place that feels secure—away from danger, but with good visibility to spot any new threats. For most people, this means we tend to position our bed away from doors and windows, but still within sight of these access points.

Creating a sense of calm and safety is bound to help you relax—a great first step toward a good night's sleep—so it's worth checking whether your bed is set up to encourage this sense of security.

FENG SHUI BALANCE

The idea that safe and relaxing places are best for sleep is echoed in the ancient Chinese practice of feng shui, which focuses on promoting a positive flow of energy known as "chi" by creating "balance." According to contemporary feng shui, the bed should be in what is called a "command position"—diagonally across from the door, not in line with it, but so the door can still be seen. The head of the bed should be against a wall, both for stability and so you can be sure there's nothing lurking behind you as you sleep—again meeting our primal need to stay safe from predators.

MAGNETIC FIELD

There is a widespread belief that your sleeping position in relation to the earth's magnetic field can also affect sleep. Ayurveda, the ancient Indian system of medicine, holds that sleeping with your head pointing northward creates a clash of positively charged energy that disrupts sleep. However, there's little scientific evidence to back this up—in fact, some studies have shown that sleeping in a north-south position, aligned with the earth's magnetic field, leads to better and deeper slumber than the east-west position that Ayurveda recommends.

If you struggle with poor sleep, it's unlikely that the position of your bed is the main cause. In addition to moving your bed, ensuring that your bedroom is a calm, inviting place that you find relaxing (see pages 170–171) is likely to be a more effective way of guaranteeing a good night's rest.

Optimum position?

Placing the bed in a north-south alignment, away from windows and doors but angled so that you still have sight of them, may help your primal brain feel safe enough to drift into slumber.

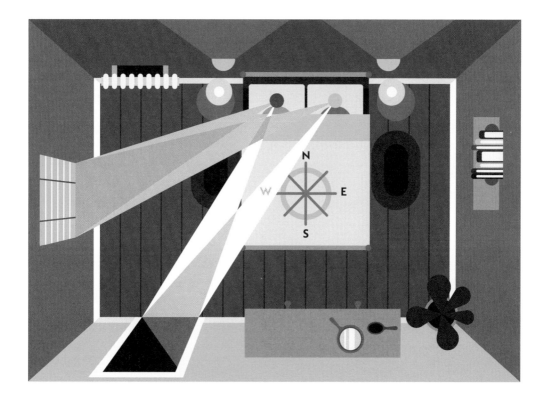

Should I sleep with the window open or closed?

There are plenty of benefits to sleeping with an open window, but some downsides, too. The choice depends on an individual's needs and circumstances.

We know that being cool helps you sleep better, so opening the window in summer will improve overall sleep quality (although bear in mind that in a hot climate, an open window could actually raise room temperature).

The atmosphere in a bedroom can quickly get stale and polluted, as the air trapped between the covers and the body is recirculated. This has been shown to interfere with sleep, so creating an airflow by opening the window can really help, especially in a small room. Air and change your bedding regularly, too, to help dispel staleness.

Also, as we breathe out carbon dioxide over the course of the night, the level of the gas in the room will rise and remain high if the window is closed. Although this isn't at all dangerous to health, one study found that with lower levels of carbon dioxide in the bedroom, people reported that the air "felt" fresher, they slept better, and they were less sleepy and more able to concentrate the next day.

WHEN TO KEEP IT SHUT

An open window can make some allergies, such as hayfever, worse and affect sleep. Also, some people find sleeping with a window open gives them a sore throat or neck pain. This might be due to a draft triggering torticollis—a muscle spasm in the neck. Heat treatment and/or massage can effectively relieve symptoms. If any of these conditions apply to you, or if it's simply not safe to leave windows open in your neighborhood, keeping the bedroom door open as you sleep will still improve air flow and help you sleep better.

An open window can improve sleep quality by up to

50%

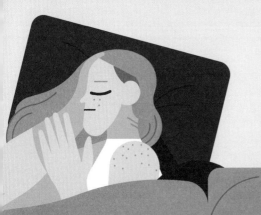
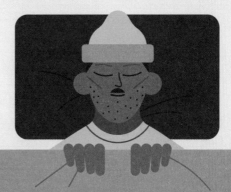
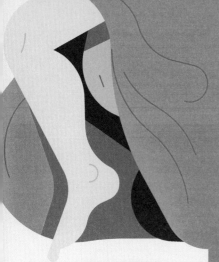

What's the ideal temperature for my bedroom?

Although the body can self-regulate its temperature to an extent, the external environment plays a significant role in either promoting or hampering good sleep. Studies show that the ideal bedroom temperature for sleep is lower than we might think—being too warm prevents the release of sleep-inducing hormones. Good ventilation is also key; opening a window (see opposite page) is often the best and cheapest way to regulate temperature, except in extreme climates. In summer, change to a lighter comforter or blanket and consider using a fan, air conditioning, or a dehumidifier to cool and circulate the air.

BLOWING HOT AND COLD

It's common for sleeping partners to prefer different bedroom temperatures, and striking a balance is down to trial and error. Research shows that women tend to feel the cold more than men, probably linked to typically higher levels of estrogen. Also, core temperature may fluctuate at different points in their menstrual cycle.

If this is your problem, it's generally better to set the bedroom at the cooler temperature, as it's easier for the "cold" partner to get cozy than it is for the "hot" person to cool down enough to sleep. You can also use separate covers with different tog ratings, a dual-control electric blanket that allows you to heat only one side of the bed, or a chill pad that lets you cool one side down.

The ideal bedroom temperature for adults is

61–64°F (16–18°C)

What should I wear in bed?

Research shows that body temperature has a significant impact on the quality of sleep—and your choice of sleepwear can make a difference.

Your temperature affects both your ability to get to and stay asleep (see pages 76–77): close-fitting clothing can raise your body temperature, blocking the signal to send you to sleep. Once asleep, being too hot or cold may cause you to wake. Nightwear in breathable fabrics such as cotton or bamboo can help regulate your temperature as you sleep.

Nightwear should not feel restrictive or uncomfortable as you move around. If this is an issue for you, sleeping naked may be the most relaxing and comfortable option. However, for others, getting into nightwear is a ritual that signals bedtime and creates positive associations.

UNDERWEAR PROS AND CONS

If you sleep in underwear, avoid tight-fitting briefs, as they create a warm microclimate in an area that prefers to be cool. In terms of reproductive health, loose-fitting boxer shorts help men maintain a healthy sperm count. Some people wear a bra in bed for comfort or because they believe it will prevent sagging, but studies suggest that this makes no difference to the tone of breast tissue.

Wearing socks in bed can lower blood pressure, which in turn helps the body prepare for sleep. A recent study showed that wearing socks in a cool room is beneficial for sleep. Participants' core body temperature remained stable and they found it easier to fall and stay asleep.

" "

In a study, wearing bed socks in a cool room led to **32** minutes' more sleep.

Should I let my pet sleep on my bed?

Whether to share your bed with your pet is a question of balancing the emotional benefits with any physical and practical drawbacks.

There is no doubt that dogs and cats provide comfort and a sense of security, and physical proximity to pets has proven benefits. The vibrations of a cat's purr range from 25–150 megahertz—frequencies that are used in ultrasound therapies to heal bone and soft tissues. And sleep specialists say that emotional support dogs can help in treating nightmares and other anxiety-related sleep disturbance in PTSD sufferers.

" "

Feeding the cat just before your bedtime may help prevent it from disturbing you at night.

SLEEPING COMPANIONS

A study found that people sleeping with one dog in the bedroom (but not on the bed) maintained good sleep efficiency (the amount of time spent asleep). However, if the dog slept on the bed, sleep was mildly disrupted.

The size and number of pets matters, too—cats are small, but they're often more active at night and may wake you if they want to go out, play, or eat.

Light sleepers or those with allergies should avoid sleeping with pets. If your partner is not eager to share the bed with a pet, keep in mind that arguments release sleep-busting stress hormones. Your own pet's sleeping habits may also affect yours. Research has shown that dogs who are stressed, bored, or lonely sleep worse than active, happy dogs—and their nocturnal restlessness may in turn disturb you.

What, if anything, should I listen to in bed?

Lullabies and bedtime stories have long been used to soothe babies and children to sleep. Podcasts, customized music playlists, and sleep apps are the adult versions of these time-honored techniques. Research shows that listening to some types of content as you fall asleep helps slow the heart and breathing, lowers blood pressure, and relaxes muscles. However, the key to success lies in choosing your material wisely.

- **Go slow.** Music or speech with a tempo of 60–80 beats per minute (BPM) that roughly mimics the human resting heart rate is proven to induce physical and mental calm. Look online for websites that list the BPM of well-known pieces of classical and popular music.

After choosing something to listen to, turn the screen face down to avoid distractions

Earbuds are more comfortable to fall asleep with

- **Go low.** The majority of listeners report that a deep, relaxed voice is the one most likely to lull them to sleep. Podcasts offering adult bedtime stories typically feature a warm, baritone voice recounting a series of slow-paced, meandering stories or articles.

- **Avoid overstimulation.** Ensure your chosen content isn't too energizing; just before bed is definitely not the time to listen to dance music, a controversial debate, or a side-splitting comedy.

TOO MUCH OF A GOOD THING?

When you find a podcast or music that helps, it's natural to rely on it to put you to sleep. However, your response diminishes a little with every exposure, and the content can become less effective over time. If you start to fear that your trusty sleep aid won't work, this can lead to anxiety or worsen an existing condition.

If this is an issue for you, CBTI (see pages 132–133), either online or face-to-face, can help you work out ways to reduce your reliance on external tools for sleep.

APP TYPES

- **De-stressors** Apps offering guided meditations and visualizations or self-hypnosis help the body and brain relax. Journaling apps can help you process thoughts before bed.

- **Background noise** Apps that play white or pink noise can help cancel out annoying, sleep-disrupting sounds around you, such as street noise. See pages 188–189 for more on this.

- **Natural sounds** Ambient noises from nature, such as rainfall, ocean waves, or rustling leaves, have a consistent, predictable rhythm that is profoundly soothing for the brain. They help lower your stress response, relaxing you for sleep.

Slip into silence

Most smartphones and apps allow you to set a time limit on listening. Start by setting your content to play for 15–20 minutes—you can lengthen the playing time if you find you're still awake when the device goes to sleep.

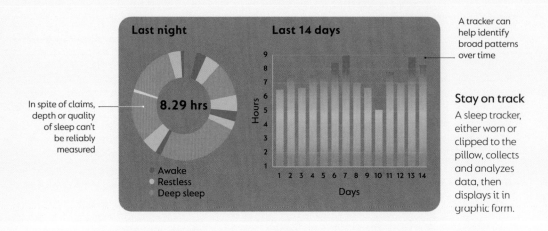

Last night

Last 14 days

8.29 hrs

- Awake
- Restless
- Deep sleep

Hours

Days

In spite of claims, depth or quality of sleep can't be reliably measured

A tracker can help identify broad patterns over time

Stay on track

A sleep tracker, either worn or clipped to the pillow, collects and analyzes data, then displays it in graphic form.

Do sleep trackers work?

Sleep-tracking devices have come a long way, but the quality of the data they capture—and their addictive qualities—are concerning for some sleep scientists. Sleep trackers record when you fall asleep and wake up and how much time you spend sleeping. Some claim to measure how long you spend in each sleep phase, but none work as well as a polysomnogram—the diagnostic tool used in the controlled environment of a sleep clinic. For instance, a tracker can easily misinterpret movements during the lightest phases of sleep as you being awake.

A tracker can be a useful guide to helping you establish a consistent routine—the key to good sleep—but you need to have a reasonable mindset about the data. It's all too easy to become obsessed with the numbers, and this anxious quest for perfection has been identified as a sleep disorder in itself: orthosomnia, where obsession with sleep data actually makes a sleep problem worse. The best tracker is your own body; the most reliable indication of a good night's sleep is whether you feel refreshed and energized when you wake.

Will reading before bed harm my sleep?

For many people, bedtime reading is one of life's great pleasures. If you find it difficult to unwind and switch off at bedtime, a good book could be your best friend. There are plenty of advantages to being a bedtime bookworm—reading before sleep is proven to reduce anxiety and stress. Research also shows that you're more likely to retain information that you read just before sleep, so reading before you close your eyes for the night can help you simultaneously relax, learn, and improve your memory. For those with insomnia, reading as part of a wind-down routine can help reduce the stimulating hormone cortisol and boost the chances of good rest.

• **Reading in bed.** For most people, this won't impact your sleep. However, if you have insomnia, it's best to read in another room and only get into bed when you are sure you're ready to sleep.

• **Print or digital?** Printed books come out on top—one study showed that 30 minutes of reading a light-emitting e-book increased the time taken to fall asleep by 10 minutes, compared to reading a printed copy.

• **Read, don't browse.** Scrolling through social media or scanning news websites doesn't count as reading—it's too stimulating and potentially stressful. Reading an absorbing narrative allows body and mind to slow down.

• **Fact or fiction?** Fiction seems to be the most sleep-friendly choice, as long as the story's not scary or emotionally harrowing.

68%

The reported reduction in stress after just six minutes of sustained reading, according to one study

Why does the slightest noise wake me up but not my partner?

Research suggests that environmental noise may affect our sleep quality more than we realize. But some people are also naturally more sound-sensitive while sleeping. In general, noise is most likely to wake us up during light Stage-2 sleep, which accounts for around half your total night's sleep. Children and older adults are more vulnerable to having their sleep disturbed by sounds.

Before and during sleep, the brain reduces its responsiveness to environmental stimuli such as noise and light. The thalamus—the sensory relay center and sleep gatekeeper—filters these out. This area of the brain also produces "sleep spindles," a type of high-frequency brainwave occurring in short bursts that determine your brain's soundproofing to external noise. A key study showed that people who produce more sleep spindles were better at tolerating increasingly loud noises—such as a phone ringing—before waking up.

"K-complex" brainwaves are another type of activity that occur before and after sleep spindles are produced and are thought to suppress the brain's arousal in response

Sleep soundproofing
Both K-complex and sleep spindles seem to play a role in reducing sensitivity to sound: K-complex firing occurs in response to external stimuli, whereas sleep spindles appear to fire in order to prevent you from being able to hear such stimuli.

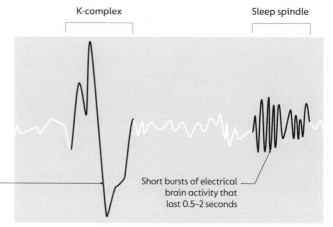

K-complex

Sleep spindle

Spontaneous burst of electrical brain activity lasting around 1 second

Short bursts of electrical brain activity that last 0.5–2 seconds

to sound. Some people produce more of these noise-blocking brainwaves than others—mainly due to genetics. However, people may also have personal "trigger" sounds that are more likely to disturb their sleep; one study of new mothers showed they were more easily woken up by their baby crying than an alarm clock.

BLOCKING OUT NOISE

• **Extra pillows, rugs,** and heavy curtains in the bedroom all help absorb noise energy and dull sound. If street noise is an issue, move your bed away from an outside wall.

• **Earplugs** have been shown to improve deep sleep. Soft foam versions are more comfortable, but all earplugs can cause wax build-up. Noise-canceling earbuds and headphones are good alternatives and can also be used to play relaxing sounds.

SLEEP-FRIENDLY SOUNDS

Many people use a sound machine or "white noise" app for a short time or throughout the night to help them fall and stay asleep. Sound, like brainwaves, is measured by frequencies in hertz. Different sound frequencies are described as noise and are allocated various colors, such as white or pink. In theory, the mixed frequencies of a consistent humming background noise (similar to a fan) help mask sudden, intrusive sounds. However, findings on white noise's effectiveness vary widely. "Pink" noise sounds gentler because the higher-pitched elements are softened. Research is limited, although a small study of older people found it improved the type of brain activity associated with deep sleep.

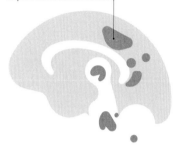

No spindles
The brain's sound-processing areas are still active and respond to external noises

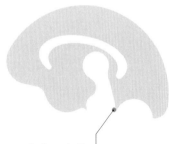

During spindles
The brain's sound-processing areas are isolated from external noises, meaning you are less likely to wake

Sleep spindle activity

Brain imaging shows how activity in the thalamus and primary auditory cortex—the areas responsible for processing sound—is reduced during sleep spindle activity in NREM sleep.

What's the best alarm?

The body's natural circadian rhythm is the ideal wake-up call; however, many of us have to rely on artificial methods to pull us out of sleep in the morning. Although some people are biologically primed to leap out of bed the moment their eyes open (see pages 78–79), in a major study, around 80 percent of people used an alarm clock on work days, and nearly 70 percent slept at least an hour longer on free days.

A loud, blaring alarm may seem like an obvious choice, especially if you need be up and ready to go quickly— but the repeated shock of such a sudden noise could eventually train your brain to anticipate it and lead to disturbed early-morning sleep.

CHOOSE A SONG

An alarm with melodic sound may have a more energizing effect than a harsh "beep beep." One study of reactions to various sounds found that melodies with rising and falling tones seemed to increase people's arousal and cognition, helping them feel less groggy. As well as melody, rhythm also seemed to affect the alertness of participants. While noting that further work is needed, researchers suggested songs such as "Good Vibrations" by The Beach Boys and "Close To Me" by The Cure were most effective in the transition from sleep to alertness.

Whatever sound you choose, avoid getting into the habit of hitting the snooze button, which can leave you feeling sluggish for longer (see page 150). Place your sound alarm device just far enough away from the bed so you have to get out of bed to turn it off—some phone-based alarm apps make you solve a puzzle or vigorously shake the phone before turning off.

An alternative to sound alarms, a dawn simulator or "sunrise alarm" gradually increases artificial light into the bedroom in the final 30–60 minutes of sleep. The theory is that this helps you wake up naturally and effectively, even when it's dark outside. In one study, people who normally found it difficult to wake up said they felt more alert and showed faster reaction times after using a sunrise alarm. The light from these alarms is much less intense than from light boxes, which are a recognized therapy for sleep disorders such as SAD (see pages 172–173). But there's some evidence that sunrise alarms can be of help to those with mild or moderate winter depression.

Using a sunrise alarm
Even through closed eyes, photoreceptor cells in the retinas can still detect light and will signal the master clock in the brain that it's time to wake up.

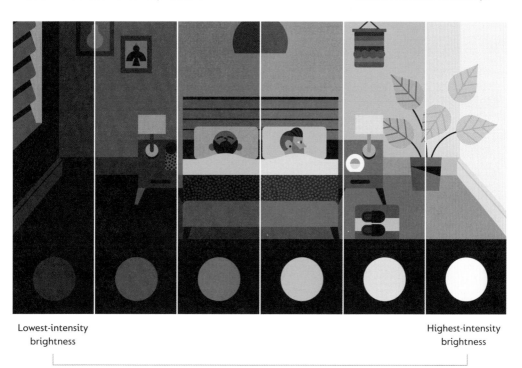

Lowest-intensity brightness

Highest-intensity brightness

7 a.m.

Brightness intensifies over 30 minutes

7:30 a.m.

Should my partner and I go to bed at the same time?

Whether you're comforting a sleepless child, catching up on work emails, or winding down with a TV series, there are plenty of reasons for staying up after your partner heads to bed.

Many people gain a deep sense of comfort and security from falling asleep next to their significant other. This isn't just physical; it can reduce stress and make you feel more emotionally connected and content with the relationship. One study found couples with mismatched sleep patterns reported more marital conflict; another suggested a link between a similar sleeping pattern and how positive people felt about their partner the next day.

However, going to bed at the same time doesn't work for everyone, and some couples find they have to stagger sleep times. In some instances, one partner may find it easier to go to bed solo and be asleep when the other partner comes to bed—for instance, if they suffer from insomnia or if the other partner snores or grinds their teeth. The priority is for both partners to get enough consistent, restorative sleep to feel fully rested.

BIRDS AND OWLS

Some people never feel sleepy at the same time as their partner because they are very different chronotypes— your biological chronotype dictates the personal peaks and troughs of your sleep/wake cycle (see pages 78–79).

If you and your partner are polar-opposite chronotypes, you could very well find yourselves at odds trying to keep the same bedtime. But most people fall somewhere in between, which should make it easier to find compromises that ensure you both get the intimacy you want and the sleep you need.

MAKING SLEEP DIFFERENCES WORK

• Talk openly about each other's sleep needs— understanding your chronotypes will help prevent hurt feelings.

• Consider hacks so you don't wake your partner by coming to bed late or rising early, such as using a night light or undressing in the bathroom.

• If being together at bedtime doesn't work, make time earlier in the evening where you can talk, cuddle, or simply enjoy being together.

" " _____

In a study of couples, those
who slept in the same bed
got around **10%** more
REM sleep, and their sleep
was less disrupted.

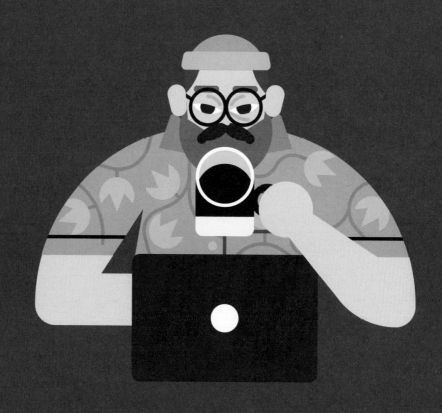

When sleep goes wrong

We constantly hear about the dire consequences of poor sleep. While it's true that good sleep and good health go hand-in-hand, there are plenty of ways to improve or resolve sleep problems, even those that are entrenched.

Can chronic sleep deprivation harm my overall health?

There's no way to sugar-coat the pill: without good sleep, the body misses out on many of its essential processes. Sleep is the body's repair shop, maintaining immunity, cleaning up the brain, and ensuring we are ready to go again when the sun rises. Most adults need between seven and nine hours of sleep a night; however, a US survey found that nearly one-third of people sleep for less than six hours.

MENTAL, EMOTIONAL, AND PHYSICAL EFFECTS

If you are constantly sleep-deprived, your ability to recall information or focus is impaired. Without enough deep sleep, the ability to learn, make decisions, and cope with stress is reduced. Evidence shows that fatigue related to sleep loss often plays a part in workplace and driving accidents. Inadequate sleep weakens our body systems. It exhausts the body—at a cellular level, the body doesn't get a chance to repair itself. Evidence shows that less than six hours of sleep a night on an ongoing basis increases the risk of developing a range of medical conditions. Lack of sleep is also a key reason why some people are less physically active, smoke, or drink excess alcohol.

RECOVERY SLEEP

Despite these harmful effects, if you prioritize sleep, your body will seize the chance to reverse the impact of sleep loss. Finding ways to increase your overall sleep time will reap huge benefits. To recoup long-term sleep loss, try going to bed 15–30 minutes earlier every night—this is not recommended if you suffer from insomnia. Naps and occasionally sleeping in can also help increase overall sleep time, although trying to claw back more than five hours in one go will likely leave you feeling groggy and may negatively affect your ongoing sleep.

AM I SLEEP-DEPRIVED?

Look out for any warning signs that you may need to increase your regular quota of sleep.

- **Physical symptoms** include tension headaches, jaw clenching or teeth grinding, irritable bowel syndrome, high blood pressure, or sexual dysfunction.

- **Psychological impact** may be irritability, impatience, memory lapses, and poor performance, as well as anxiety and depression.

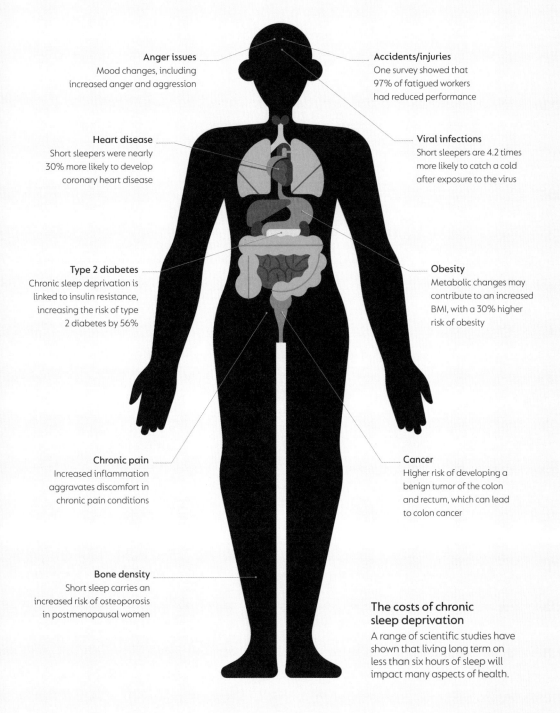

Anger issues
Mood changes, including increased anger and aggression

Accidents/injuries
One survey showed that 97% of fatigued workers had reduced performance

Heart disease
Short sleepers were nearly 30% more likely to develop coronary heart disease

Viral infections
Short sleepers are 4.2 times more likely to catch a cold after exposure to the virus

Type 2 diabetes
Chronic sleep deprivation is linked to insulin resistance, increasing the risk of type 2 diabetes by 56%

Obesity
Metabolic changes may contribute to an increased BMI, with a 30% higher risk of obesity

Chronic pain
Increased inflammation aggravates discomfort in chronic pain conditions

Cancer
Higher risk of developing a benign tumor of the colon and rectum, which can lead to colon cancer

Bone density
Short sleep carries an increased risk of osteoporosis in postmenopausal women

The costs of chronic sleep deprivation
A range of scientific studies have shown that living long term on less than six hours of sleep will impact many aspects of health.

I've always had sleep issues. What's wrong with me?

Consistently struggling to get to or stay asleep or waking too early are the classic hallmarks of insomnia—a sleep disorder with far-reaching effects.

Anyone who has experienced insomnia knows all too well the numerous effects it can have on daily life: daytime drowsiness, irritability, poor memory, fatigue, and difficulties in relationships can all follow on from this condition. Studies have indicated that insomnia affects approximately 10–30 percent of the population worldwide, with rates as high as 60 percent in some countries. Women and older people seem to be particularly susceptible.

Insomnia progression

This graphic shows that insomnia usually begins with a triggering event. Sometimes there are latent risk factors before the onset, too. To cope with the stressful trigger, you may develop unhelpful behaviors that actually maintain insomnia. If these behaviors become ingrained, they can mean chronic insomnia develops.

WHAT CAUSES INSOMNIA?

A combination of psychological, behavioral, environmental, and biological components are all thought to play their part in the onset and continuance

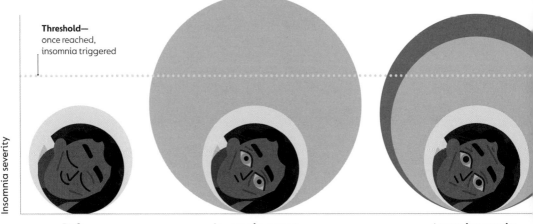

Threshold— once reached, insomnia triggered

Insomnia severity

Before
Underlying risk factors, like having anxiety, make it more likely insomnia will develop

Insomnia onset
A stressful trigger, such as a death in the family, means insomnia threshold is reached

Acute insomnia
You begin to behave in unhelpful ways that perpetuate insomnia—for example, too much caffeine

of insomnia. Some people have a higher risk of developing insomnia: among the predisposing factors are anxiety, depression, some prescription medications, chronic stress, or some of the hormonal changes that come with age. Studies have also shown that genetics play a part, and insomnia often runs in families.

Specific life events can also disrupt sleep and trigger a bout of insomnia, such as the stress of a new job, as well as changes to schedules caused by shift work or jet lag. A few bad nights of sleep here and there is normal, and acute, or short-term, insomnia often disappears once the stressful event passes or we adapt to it. However, for some people, insomnia can become chronic, or long-term. Once someone has had difficulty sleeping for more than four weeks, they have usually begun to think about sleep differently, acting in ways that perpetuate the issue. Behaviors that contribute to insomnia continuing include caffeine, alcohol, or nicotine use; inconsistent bedtimes; and too much time spent browsing social media in bed.

INSOMNIA IS A HUNGRY BEAST

When insomnia strikes, changing your bedtime habits, developing relaxation strategies, and practicing good sleep hygiene are vital. Early intervention in these areas can often be enough to stop insomnia from becoming chronic. It's also important to remind yourself that a bout of acute insomnia is perfectly normal; insomnia is fed by fear, so the more you worry about not being able to sleep, the worse it is likely to get. CBTI (see pages 132–133) is one of the most effective techniques for helping you rethink things and address your bad habits and negative thoughts around sleep. By doing so, you can learn to nurture the mental and physical conditions necessary for a good night's sleep.

KEY

- Underlying risk factors
- Specific life event triggers
- Behaviors that maintain insomnia

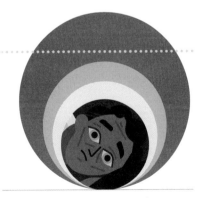

Chronic insomnia

If unhelpful behaviors are not addressed, even if initial stressor passes, insomnia becomes chronic

Does lack of sleep impair judgment?

We're often advised to sleep on a big decision, and science bears out this piece of folk wisdom.

Our sleep has a profound effect on the way we process information. Because the brain is so complex and interconnected, this is a difficult area to research, and scientific findings vary—as do individual sleep needs. Research shows that going for only 17 hours without sleep can impair cognitive performance (including reaction time) nearly as much as being at some countries' legal alcohol limit for driving.

Neuroscientists do know that insufficient sleep has a particular impact on the brain's prefrontal cortex, the area that enables us to problem-solve, reason, organize, plan, and perform other higher cognitive tasks. The medial prefrontal cortex, which also acts to regulate emotions, may be less able to "talk down" the amygdala, which processes feelings (especially fear), reacts to stress, and triggers the body's "fight-or-flight" stress response. Sufficient sleep is essential for efficient storage of the

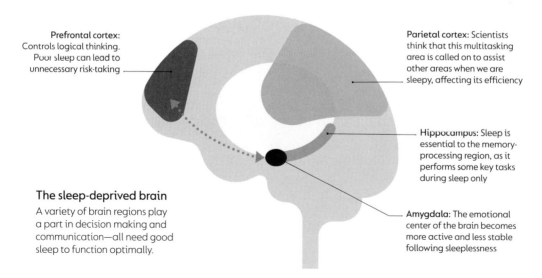

Prefrontal cortex: Controls logical thinking. Poor sleep can lead to unnecessary risk-taking

Parietal cortex: Scientists think that this multitasking area is called on to assist other areas when we are sleepy, affecting its efficiency

Hippocampus: Sleep is essential to the memory-processing region, as it performs some key tasks during sleep only

Amygdala: The emotional center of the brain becomes more active and less stable following sleeplessness

The sleep-deprived brain
A variety of brain regions play a part in decision making and communication—all need good sleep to function optimally.

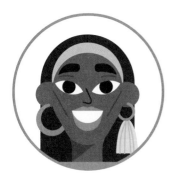

Well-rested people interpreted the expression correctly

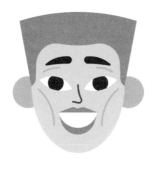

Participants were asked to judge the mood of the person in an image

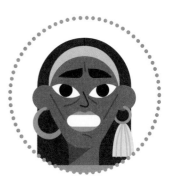

Sleep-deprived people interpreted the expression wrongly

information that may help you make decisions: the brain consolidates different types of learned information into memories during the different stages and cycles of sleep (see pages 54–55). Sleep loss may also hamper cognitive flexibility—the ability to rapidly adjust to new information or changing events. Not only does poor sleep impair your thought processes, but there's evidence that it also prevents you from recognizing that your thinking might be impaired. One study found sleep-deprived participants tended to claim that they were still functioning well—even when tests showed their cognitive abilities had significantly declined.

THE MORNING AFTER

In daily life, the cognitive consequences of a poor night's sleep will usually only cause us minor irritation. Sometimes, however, lives depend on sharp and accurate judgment; the US space shuttle *Challenger* fell to earth after a postlaunch explosion, killing its crew. An official report found some key managers got less than two hours' sleep the night before, and sleep loss and early morning shift work contributed to some poor decisions.

Misreading the signs

Sleep-deprived people tend to see the world in a more negative light. In one study, participants were shown a series of images of people with different expressions. Sleep-deprived individuals consistently attributed more negative emotions to the faces than well-rested participants.

201

What's the minimum amount of sleep I need to function well?

The base amount of sleep you need is personal to you and will depend on a variety of factors, including your age, health, activity, and stress levels.

As a general guide, adults require between seven and nine hours' sleep a night for the brain and body to perform all the necessary biological tasks that can only happen during sleep. Just a few nights of four hours' sleep has been shown to negatively affect heart rate, blood pressure, mood, and memory—although effects are reversed when you start sleeping normally again. Although many people report that they function well on five or six hours' sleep a night, that fact is that most will be chronically sleep-deprived.

AM I A TRUE SHORT SLEEPER?

A few people—thought to be less than 1 percent globally—are naturally able to thrive on less sleep due to a quirk in their genetic code. A gene mutation, named DEC2, appears to work by making it easier for the body to produce more orexin, which wakes us up and keeps us alert. Studies show that people with this mutation are able to sleep for around six hours with no impact on their daytime performance. Research also found that the family members of short sleepers had another rare genetic mutation called ADRB1, which affects their sleep/wake cycle.

Although there is no widely available test to confirm if you are genetically a short sleeper, if you tend to be highly active and efficient, feel well rested in the morning, and have relatives with similar traits, it could be that you are a member of this exclusive club.

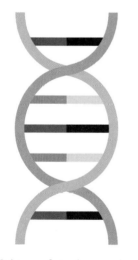

Science of staying awake
Since the discovery of the first "short-sleep gene" in 2009, researchers have identified two further mutations that may also enable natural short sleep.

CAN I SLEEP TOO MUCH?

Around 2 percent of people are affected by "hypersomnia"—they may need as much as 10–12 hours' sleep every night and still feel sleepy and nap in the daytime. This excessive sleeping has many different causes, some of which are genetic; it can also be a side effect of prescription medication or a symptom of depression. Specific sleep disorders that shorten or disrupt nighttime sleep may also prompt sufferers to spend extra daytime hours in bed to compensate.

While research findings vary, there is some evidence that habitual oversleeping may be as detrimental to health as too little sleep. Studies have found that both can be associated with a higher risk of developing certain conditions (see below).

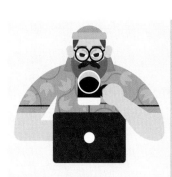

Too little sleep:

- Reduced reasoning skills
- Higher risk of obesity due to hunger and overeating
- Higher risk of heart disease and strokes
- Possible risk factor for dementia

less than **6**
hours' sleep

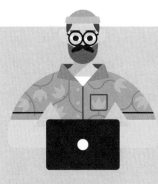

Ideal amount of sleep

- Many scientific studies have identified seven to nine hours' sleep as the optimum length of sleep to maintain physical and mental health in the vast majority of adults

7–9
hours' sleep

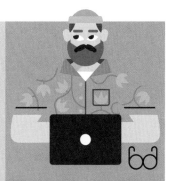

Too much sleep:

- Reduced reasoning ability
- Links to faster cognitive decline
- Higher risk of heart disease and strokes
- Possible early warning sign of dementia

more than **9**
hours' sleep

What are microsleeps?

Sitting in a long, boring meeting, your head suddenly lolls to one side and you jerk back to reality. This is a microsleep—a brief, involuntary bout of unconsciousness. You may not even be aware of a microsleep, but under research conditions, your brainwave activity would clearly indicate that you were asleep with your senses switched off and unresponsive to the world around you. Microsleeps don't always mean we close our eyes—so if you've seen someone's eyes glaze over and they start to look zoned out, they could well be having a microsleep in front of you.

WHAT CAUSES MICROSLEEPS?

When we are fully rested, the pressure to sleep is low for most of the day and our "sleep switch" stays off. However, when we have not had sufficient sleep, that pressure stays high and can peak at any time. As soon as the body senses a slowing down (for instance, when we zone out in that tedious meeting), it seizes the opportunity and flips the sleep switch, and it's lights out for a moment.

Sleep deprivation is the main cause of microsleeps, with shift workers—especially those with changeable shift patterns, such as medical professionals—most at risk. Sleep disorders that disrupt sleep, such as narcolepsy or sleep apnea, can also be a factor.

The only way to eliminate microsleeps is to tackle the cause of your sleep deprivation. When that's not possible—for instance, when you have a newborn baby—try to claw back sleep whenever you can (such as napping whenever your baby does) and be assured that you will weather this temporary sleep drought without long-term harm to your health.

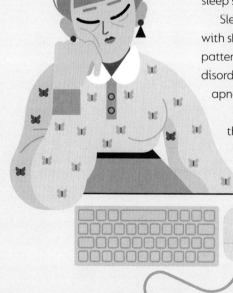

How dangerous is driving when I'm tired?

Have you ever felt your eyes starting to close when driving? If so, you are not alone. Drowsy driving is surprisingly common and a major cause of accidents. Drive when you are drowsy, and the impact on your performance is similar to being under the influence of drugs or alcohol: your judgment is impaired, reactions are slower, and you can even fail to spot hazards. Driving drowsy also increases your risk of falling into a microsleep at the wheel (see opposite page), especially when you're on a long, monotonous drive. Even the briefest loss of consciousness can be catastrophic, so the advice is simple: never drive when you're tired.

20%
of accidents on interstate highways and divided highways in the UK are sleep-related

ARE YOU AT RISK?

You are most at risk of drowsy driving if you are currently suffering from chronic sleep deprivation or sleep apnea; a shift worker; or driving at night. However, just one night of disrupted sleep can impact your alertness. If you're tired, think carefully before you get behind the wheel—opening the windows or turning up the music is not going to counter that irresistible urge to close your eyes. Stop driving as soon as you can if you experience any of the following:

- Yawning
- Heavy eyelids
- Difficulty concentrating
- Missing a turn
- Drifting across lanes or hitting a rumble strip

Don't start driving again until you've had proper rest (see box, left). No matter how inconvenient it may be to interrupt your journey, there's no alternative. Driving drowsy is risking your own and everyone else's safety.

CAFFEINE-KICK DRIVING HACK

The best temporary fix for fatigue is a cup of strong coffee, followed by a 30-minute nap. The caffeine in coffee takes around 30 minutes to kick in, so it will reach its full power just as you wake.

If I don't get enough sleep, will I get Alzheimer's disease?

Growing evidence suggests that sleep can protect against Alzheimer's disease and dementia, but overblown headlines proclaiming that a bad night's sleep causes Alzheimer's have fueled widespread anxiety.

The study that triggered the headlines identified the role of a protein called beta-amyloid in neurodegeneration—the progressive loss of function of nerve cells. Beta-amyloid builds up naturally in the brain but is found in abnormally large amounts in those with Alzheimer's. When beta-amyloid accumulates, it forms clumps, known as plaques, that disrupt the nutrient supply to brain cells. This kills the cells and in turn causes neurodegeneration and destroys memory. This study found that those who experienced a night of sleep deprivation had slightly higher than normal levels of beta-amyloid, leading the researchers to suggest a possible link between poor sleep and Alzheimer's.

A PROTEIN CALLED TAU

More recent research has shown that tau, another protein found in brain neurons, may play a more significant role in the relationship between sleep and Alzheimer's. Abnormal tau clusters, known as tangles, have been found in the brains of Alzheimer's patients, and sleep deprivation appears to cause tau to increase. This is likely to be because during Stage-3 deep sleep, the brain prompts the release of cerebrospinal fluid (CSF). CSF is thought to help flush toxins through the brain's glymphatic system—including beta-amyloid and tau—and disrupted sleep may therefore mean missing out on this vital clearance process. It isn't yet clear whether simply having high levels of beta-amyloid or tau increases the risk of Alzheimer's onset—research is ongoing—but what we do know is that poor sleep is likely to be only one piece in solving the Alzheimer's puzzle.

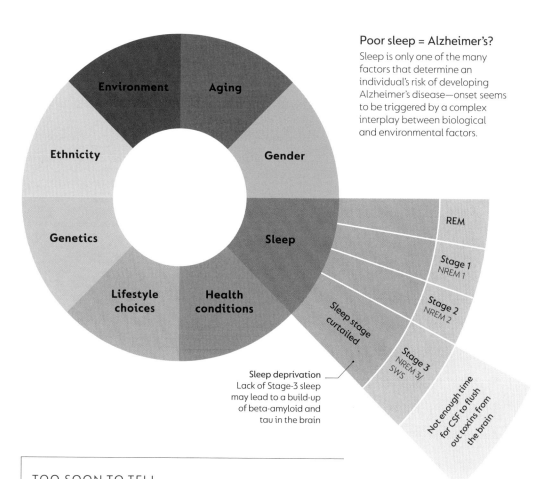

Poor sleep = Alzheimer's?

Sleep is only one of the many factors that determine an individual's risk of developing Alzheimer's disease—onset seems to be triggered by a complex interplay between biological and environmental factors.

Environment

Aging

Ethnicity

Gender

Genetics

Sleep

Lifestyle choices

Health conditions

REM

Sleep stage curtailed

Stage 1
NREM 1

Stage 2
NREM 2

Stage 3
NREM 3/
SWS

Not enough time for CSF to flush out toxins from the brain

Sleep deprivation
Lack of Stage-3 sleep may lead to a build-up of beta-amyloid and tau in the brain

TOO SOON TO TELL

• Even if you are regularly sleep-deprived, there's still no clear evidence that you are more at risk of developing Alzheimer's. Of course, sleeping well will certainly boost overall health and help both body and brain manage the aging process.

• The link between sleep and Alzheimer's is being intensively researched. Large-scale studies could soon tell us whether finding ways to increase Stage-3, deep, slow-wave sleep could reduce the risk of neurodegeneration.

What's the impact of long-term stress on sleep?

"Stress" means different things to different people, but biologically, it's a specific physiological response that puts our systems on high alert.

The body's stress response, known as our "fight-or-flight" response, is the activation of the sympathetic nervous system (SNS) in response to a potential threat (stressor). Once triggered, the SNS directs various changes in the body in order to equip us with enough energy and focus to react and respond to whatever threat we are facing.

THE IMPACT OF STRESS ON THE BODY

If you are stressed in response to a short-term stressor, such as a near-miss while driving, or a medium-term stressor, such as a work deadline, these are both unlikely to have a huge impact on your sleep. When a stressor is present long term, things may become problematic—for both sleep and general health and well-being.

The stress hormone cortisol also plays a vital role in our sleep/wake cycle (see pages 26–27), naturally decreasing at night so we can get to sleep, then rising in the morning to wake us. If the body is in a persistent state of stress, high levels of cortisol can override this natural rhythm and prevent sleep, meaning we miss out on vital rest and repair functions.

When we finally do get to sleep, we may then wake with already elevated levels of cortisol. This leaves the body trapped in a cycle of toxic stress, enduring more and more wear and tear. This can eventually lead to physical problems such as impaired immunity, an increased risk of digestive and metabolic problems, and heart attacks, as well as emotional problems such as anxiety and depression.

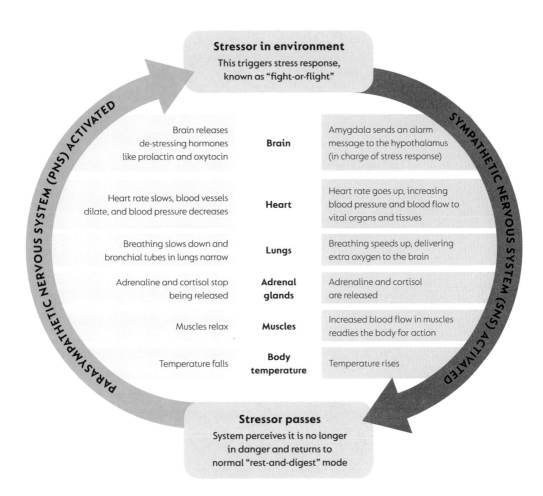

Stressor in environment
This triggers stress response, known as "fight-or-flight"

PARASYMPATHETIC NERVOUS SYSTEM (PNS) ACTIVATED

SYMPATHETIC NERVOUS SYSTEM (SNS) ACTIVATED

	Brain	
Brain releases de-stressing hormones like prolactin and oxytocin		Amygdala sends an alarm message to the hypothalamus (in charge of stress response)
Heart rate slows, blood vessels dilate, and blood pressure decreases	**Heart**	Heart rate goes up, increasing blood pressure and blood flow to vital organs and tissues
Breathing slows down and bronchial tubes in lungs narrow	**Lungs**	Breathing speeds up, delivering extra oxygen to the brain
Adrenaline and cortisol stop being released	**Adrenal glands**	Adrenaline and cortisol are released
Muscles relax	**Muscles**	Increased blood flow in muscles readies the body for action
Temperature falls	**Body temperature**	Temperature rises

Stressor passes
System perceives it is no longer in danger and returns to normal "rest-and-digest" mode

MANAGING STRESS FOR BETTER SLEEP

To be able to sleep, your body needs to dial down the SNS. The parasympathetic nervous system (PNS) is the key to this. The PNS effectively reverses the effects of high levels of cortisol experienced during times of stress, returning the body to a state of homeostasis (stable internal conditions) so it is able to move between the two systems without becoming stuck on high alert. Finding ways to successfully activate the PNS will help you manage your stress response. Key techniques that can help are relaxation strategies and gentle exercise (see pages 124–125 and 112–113).

The stress response

The SNS is initially triggered by a stressor and readies us for action; once the stressor passes, the PNS is activated to calm the stress response. If we do not perceive a stressor to have been resolved, the body remains on high alert—which can be harmful in the long term.

Why do I talk in my sleep?

Sleeptalking (also known as somniloquy) is a common parasomnia—an umbrella term for various unusual behaviors we engage in while asleep.

Sleeptalkers may mumble, groan, laugh, shout random words, or speak full sentences. One study found that the most frequently spoken word is "no," and that swear words featured 800 times more often than in an individual's daytime talk! Sleeptalking is more common in children, and most grow out of the habit as their sleep-controlling brain mechanisms mature. It's not known why, but sleeptalking is equally distributed among boys and girls, but for adults, it is more common in men.

People often assume that sleeptalking occurs when they are acting out intense, emotional dreams, but in fact sleeptalking occurs during every stage of sleep.

NO CAUSE FOR CONCERN

Sleeptalking on its own has no medical significance and doesn't require any treatment, although it may cause issues for a sleeptalker's partner. If your bedmate's midnight mutterings wake you up, wearing silicone earplugs can help. Alternatively, try placing a white- or pink-noise machine or an electric fan in the room.

Common triggers for sleeptalking in adults include stress, anxiety, depression, sleep deprivation, caffeine, alcohol, and some medications. It can also occur alongside other, more serious sleep-related problems, including sleep apnea, and seems to run in families.

If you worry that you may spill your deepest, darkest secrets while sleeptalking, rest assured that neither science nor the law considers sleeptalk to be the product of a conscious, rational mind—so anything you say is inadmissible in court!

" "

Almost **50%** of children under 10, but only **5%** of adults, talk in their sleep.

Why do I walk in my sleep?

17%
of children
regularly sleepwalk

Sleepwalking (also known as somnambulism) is another parasomnia. Like sleeptalking, it can affect people of all ages, but it is much more common in children. A range of behaviors comes under the category of sleepwalking: as well as simply wandering around, people may get dressed, move furniture around, have sex, or even try to drive a car! Episodes can last from a few seconds to around 30 minutes.

The causes of sleepwalking are not fully understood, but we do know that episodes usually occur within the first two or three hours of nodding off, just as a person enters the deepest stage of sleep. As with sleeptalkers, sleepwalkers are not acting out dreams. In common with other parasomnias, sleepwalking can be triggered by external factors—such as stress, alcohol, physical or mental illness, sleep deprivation, or an erratic sleep schedule—and also runs in families. Although there is no cure, episodes usually become fewer with age—only 2–4 percent of adults regularly sleepwalk, possibly because people experience less deep sleep as they get older.

KEEPING SLEEPWALKERS SAFE
Despite there being no direct health risk, sleepwalking can be risky, as people may put themselves in harm's way. Research also suggests that sleepwalkers may not feel pain, and many stay asleep and continue their activities even after injuring themselves.

If you or someone you live with is a sleepwalker, look for ways to reduce the risk of accidents. It's a complete myth that it's dangerous to wake a sleepwalker—the safest course of action is to gently rouse the person, reassure them, and guide them back to bed.

Why can't I stop eating at night?

Whether it's waking surrounded by food packaging with no clue how it got there or being stuck in a rut of late-night meals to get you to sleep, sleep eating disorders are relatively rare but distressing conditions. The two main sleep eating disorders are Nocturnal Sleep-Related Eating Disorder (NSRED) and Night Eating Syndrome (NES). Some professionals categorize these as eating disorders, others as parasomnias (sleep disorders with unusual behaviors), or a combination of both. Regardless, both conditions are hard to overcome alone and require professional diagnosis and treatment.

NOCTURNAL SLEEP-RELATED EATING DISORDER

It may seem implausible that someone seemingly unconscious can prepare themselves food and drink and then consume it, but this is an all-too-familiar reality for those with NSRED. More common among women, individuals usually remember little or nothing of their actions when they wake. Apart from risking obesity and type 2 diabetes, sufferers might also injure themselves while cooking or suffer an allergic reaction or choking as a result of eating unsuitable or harmful foods.

Theories on what triggers NSRED include use of certain medications, other sleep problems, a mood disorder, or sleep deprivation, which may mean that the appetite-suppressing hormone leptin isn't released as it should be during sleep (for more on leptin, see pages 86–87).

" " It's estimated that **1–3%** of adults have a sleep eating disorder.

NIGHT EATING SYNDROME

NES typically involves a person feeling compelled to eat a lot between dinner and bedtime, then waking in the night and eating again to help them return to sleep. It seems to be more common in people who may not maintain a regular eating pattern, such as students; those with highly stressful lifestyles; or people who might work straight through the day without stopping to eat. It may also be a response to crash dieting—the body signals urgently to the brain that it needs food, and the result is overeating at the worst time of day for good sleep.

Those who live with NES are often overweight, and sufferers often also struggle with issues such as depression, substance abuse, or poor self-image. Like NSRED, this condition is more prevalent in women.

SEEKING TREATMENT

People with sleep eating disorders are often reluctant to ask for help. It can take them years to seek treatment, often due to a sense of shame and a fear of being judged or not being believed. Long term, these disorders can lead to anxiety and depression, as well as weight-related health issues, so it's important to see a medical professional. These conditions are definitely treatable—medications can be helpful, as well as lifestyle changes and talking therapies to address underlying issues that may be compounding the problem.

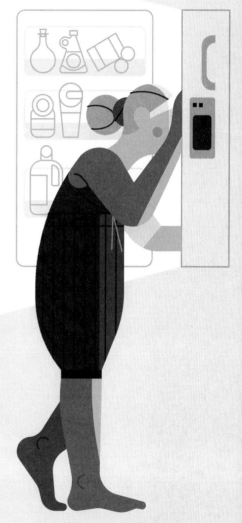

Midnight hunger
With sufferers of NES, the urge to eat builds until it peaks just before bedtime, often accompanied by low mood or increased anxiety. In the morning, their appetite is often poor.

Is lack of sleep ruining my sex life?

If you and your partner don't make love as often as you would like, it could be time to reexamine your relationship with sleep.

Sleep and sex are intimately connected; sex is good exercise and relieves mental stress, releasing "happy" endorphins and relaxing hormones. It also strengthens the bond between couple,s and when we're sleeping well, we're more likely to feel like having sex.

Exhaustion is a passion killer, though. Sleep deprivation makes it hard to find energy for anything, let alone sex, and sleep pressure (see pages 24–25) ensures that the body will often choose sleep over sex. Research shows that certain sleep disorders, such as obstructive sleep apnea, are associated with erectile dysfunction and lower sex drive.

Fatigue can also disrupt the production of the hormones testosterone and estrogen, which affect sexual desire. In a study, healthy young men saw a 10–15 percent drop in testosterone levels after a week of sleeping for five hours a night.

Lack of sleep also raises levels of the stress hormone cortisol. The "fight-or-flight" stress response redirects blood

Hormones and sex drive

The day after poor sleep, stress hormones are high and sex hormones stay low; sex is probably off the menu. However, after good rest, your libido gets a hormonal boost and your positive mood makes intimacy and sex more likely.

KEY

▬ Cortisol

▬ Testosterone

Day 1

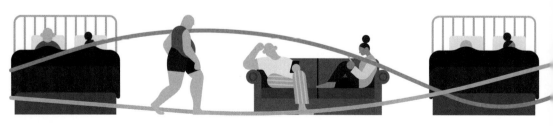

| A poor night's sleep | Tiredness causes irritability and stress | Couples less likely to connect with each other | Neither partner feels like sex |

away from sex organs, and eventually this may lower libido or lead to erectile dysfunction. One study noted that women with increased cortisol experienced lower libido and arousal.

RESET THE BALANCE

The good news is we can boost our sex lives by getting more sleep. One study found that after one extra hour of sleep, participants were 14 percent more likely to have sex the following day. To help reset your sleep–sex relationship:

• **Create a daily "wind-down hour"** Before bedtime, spend an hour relaxing together and reconnecting. Don't focus on sex at this stage; it's all about relaxation and intimacy. If you both feel mentally and physically exhausted, try a gentle 20-minute yoga or stretching routine to revive flagging energy and reconnect with your bodies.

• **Leave smartphones outside** Switch off all digital devices before your wind-down hour, and always leave smartphones outside the bedroom.

SEPARATE BEDROOMS

Research suggests that problems often occur at the same time with sleep and relationships. Some couples find that sleeping in separate bedrooms can actually improve their sex life. With each partner able to personalize their sleep space and get enough good-quality sleep, conflict may diminish. Some couples report that "date nights" in the partner's room provide added anticipation and excitement.

Day 2

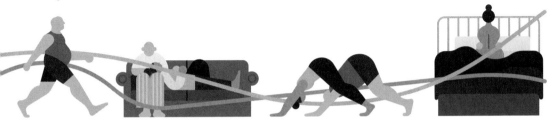

After good sleep: feeling energized and positive

Couples more likely to relax and feel intimate

Gentle exercise before bed

Couples feel in the mood for sex

I'm blind—is that why I sleep badly?

An estimated 285 million people worldwide are visually impaired in some way, and many experience significant sleep problems.

Because our 24-hour sleep/wake cycle is regulated by light, visual impairment can impact both the quantity and quality of sleep. It's a common misconception that blindness equates to absolute darkness; in fact, many blind and partially sighted people do have some light perception, which helps them synchronize their circadian rhythm to the natural 24-hour day–night cycle.

MOVABLE CYCLES

Around 10 percent of visually impaired people have no light perception, meaning that the photoreceptors in the retina that normally signal the brain to regulate the 24-hour cycle aren't stimulated. This puts them at risk of a condition known as Non-24-Hour Sleep-Wake Disorder ("Non-24"), where the internal body clock doesn't synchronize to the 24-hour day and becomes "free-running." If their natural circadian rhythm is set longer than 24 hours, a person may feel like going to sleep at midnight one day, then later the next night, and so on. If they have to get up at a certain time, the resulting build-up of sleep deprivation can lead to shorter sleep times, poor-quality sleep, excessive daytime sleepiness, and even obstructive sleep apnea. The Non-24 circadian period usually ranges from 23.8 to 25 hours.

Non-24 occurs in up to 70 percent of completely blind people. It can also occur in sighted people—long-term shift workers seem to be especially at risk. Ask your doctor about strategies for managing and treating Non-24. Melatonin therapy can be effective, but it must be prescribed by a sleep specialist to suit individual needs.

Typical 24-hour sleeping pattern

Sleep/wake pattern is kept stable by daily external cues from daylight and darkness

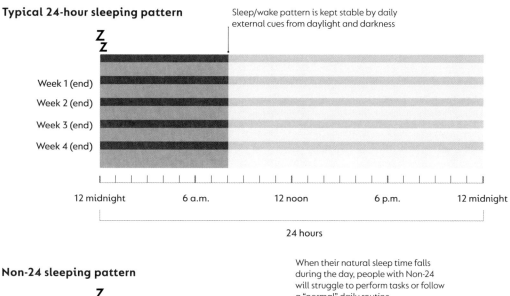

Week 1 (end)

Week 2 (end)

Week 3 (end)

Week 4 (end)

12 midnight   6 a.m.   12 noon   6 p.m.   12 midnight

24 hours

Non-24 sleeping pattern

When their natural sleep time falls during the day, people with Non-24 will struggle to perform tasks or follow a "normal" daily routine

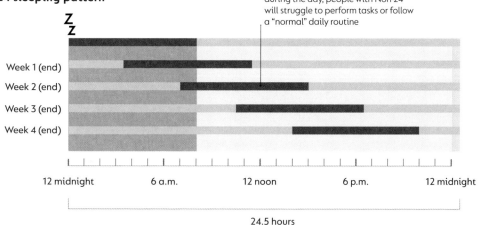

Week 1 (end)

Week 2 (end)

Week 3 (end)

Week 4 (end)

12 midnight   6 a.m.   12 noon   6 p.m.   12 midnight

24.5 hours

Shifting sleep patterns

If a visually impaired person has enough light sensitivity, their circadian rhythm will synchronize with the 24-hour day–night cycle. This keeps the timing of sleep and wake consistent (see above, top). On a body clock that runs longer than 24 hours (see above, bottom), you feel sleepy progressively later each day. Over time, your natural sleep timing drifts, eventually rotating all the way around the clock.

KEY

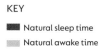

Natural sleep time

Natural awake time

Glossary

Adenosine Neurotransmitter released by the brain that creates the urge to sleep. Levels increase the longer you are awake.

Brainwaves Electrical activity in the brain. Speed and amplitude vary depending on level of consciousness and stage of sleep.

Chronotype Genetically programmed timing of your individual circadian rhythm that dictates when you tend to sleep/wake.

Circadian rhythm Natural internal biological clock that regulates the timing of various biological and behavioral changes across a 24-hour cycle.

Cognitive behavioral therapy for insomnia (CBTI) A structured treatment technique to help identify and overcome problematic thoughts and behaviors that are preventing or disrupting sleep.

Cortisol Stress hormone that increases alertness. Peaks in the morning to help us wake.

Deep sleep/slow-wave sleep (SWS) Stage-3 (NREM 3) sleep where brainwaves are slowest and it is more difficult to be roused. The most restorative type of sleep where most bodily repair processes take place.

Excessive daytime sleepiness (EDS) Also called "hypersomnia"—individuals either sleep too much or fall asleep repeatedly during the day.

Gamma-aminobutyric acid (GABA) Neurotransmitter that calms the body's stress response.

Hormones Chemical messengers that are delivered via the bloodstream and trigger certain bodily functions.

Hypnic jerk A reflex that causes involuntary muscle movements in the legs while falling asleep.

Hypothalamus Small area of the brain involved in regulation of bodily rhythms and hormone production.

Insomnia Sleep disorder characterized by difficulty falling or staying asleep, frequent waking during the night, or waking too early.

Light sleep The first two stages of sleep from which you can be easily woken: Stage-1 (NREM 1) sleep and Stage 2 (NREM 2).

Limbic system The brain's emotional response center.

Melatonin Hormone naturally produced in the pineal gland that promotes the urge to sleep.

Memory consolidation The way in which recent experiences are processed and transferred to long-term memory so they may be retrieved and recalled at a later time.

Microsleep A brief, involuntary bout of unconsciousness.

Narcolepsy A neurological disorder that causes a sudden and temporary loss of consciousness.

Neurotransmitters Chemical messengers in the brain that pass information between nerve cells.

Non-rapid eye movement (NREM) sleep The first three stages of sleep, increasing in depth as they progress.

Obstructive sleep apnea (OSA) A sleep disorder in which a person's airway repeatedly becomes blocked, causing them to stop breathing and gasp for air.

Parasomnia Umbrella term for unusual behaviors we engage in (such as sleepwalking) while asleep or in the period between sleep and wakefulness.

Parasympathetic nervous system (PNS) Branch of the autonomic nervous system that calms the body's stress response once a stressor/threat has passed.

Pineal gland Produces melatonin and regulates secretion of various other hormones.

Rapid eye movement (REM) sleep Stage of sleep in which the brain is as highly active as when we are awake. Dreaming and memory consolidation occur during this stage.

REM rebound Occurs following a period of sleep deprivation when duration of REM sleep increases in a bid to maintain your regular sleep pattern.

Serotonin Hormone involved in mood regulation; also required for the production of melatonin.

Sleep cycle Progressively passing through all four stages of sleep represents one sleep cycle. Most people experience 4–5 cycles a night.

Sleep debt Also known as sleep deficit, the difference between the amount of sleep you need versus the amount you get.

Sleep efficiency The difference between how long you spend in bed versus how long you sleep.

Sleep hygiene A series of behavioral and environmental recommendations to help improve sleep.

Sleep inertia The grogginess felt when waking suddenly from deep (SWS) or REM sleep.

Sleep pressure Also called "sleep drive" or "sleep urge." Caused by the accumulation of sleep-promoting substances in the brain over the course of the day and is only reduced by going to sleep.

Sleep stages The four distinct phases of sleep: three stages of non-REM (NREM) sleep and one stage of rapid eye movement (REM) sleep. Each stage is characterized by unique brainwave activity.

Sleep/wake cycle The 24-hour cycle of moving between the states of sleep and wakefulness.

Stress response Also known as "fight or flight." The sequence of physiological changes in the body in response to a perceived threat.

Suprachiasmatic nucleus (SCN) The body's master clock, which regulates the timing of different bodily functions. Located in the hypothalamus.

Sympathetic nervous system (SNS) Branch of the autonomic nervous system that regulates the body's stress response.

Zeitgebers External environmental cues that regulate, reset, or disrupt circadian rhythms. Cues include daylight and timing of meals.

Index

memory 15, 30, 54–55
menopause 60–61, 63
menstruation 77, 90
microsleeps 204, 205
mindfulness 124, 125
monophasic sleep 140, 141
mood 102–103
"morning larks" 78, 79, 148, 149
multivitamins 156
music 111, 184, 185

N

napping 19, 35, 45, 53, 56, 59,
    138–139, 140, 147, 150
  timing and length of nap 35,
    138–139, 143
  unhelpful 139
narcolepsy 16, 24, 52, 70, 139, 204
natural light 34, 62, 144, 164,
    173, 175
nicotine see smoking
"night owls" 78, 79, 148, 149
night terrors 47
nightmares 47, 119, 173, 185
nocturnal lagophthalmos 67
noise 35, 111, 188 189
Non-24-Hour Sleep-Wake
    Disorder 216
NREM sleep 28

O

obstructive sleep apnea (OSA)
    17, 56, 63, 69, 74, 75, 85, 87,
    94, 139, 156, 157, 159, 204,
    205, 210, 214
older people 19, 62–63
orexin 24, 52, 202

orthosomnia 186
oxytocin 26, 88, 165

P

pain, chronic 92–93, 94
parasomnias 210–211, 212
parasympathetic nervous
    system (PNS) 81, 160,
    177, 209
period gene (PER) 16, 148
periodic limb movement
    disorder (PLMD) 94
pets, sharing your bed with 183
pillows 57, 95, 96, 176
polyphasic sleep 140
polysomnography 17, 186
pregnancy 56–57, 95
probiotics 106–107, 113
progesterone 26, 56, 58, 61, 90
progressive muscle relaxation 93
prolactin 27, 59, 88, 92–93
proprioception 44, 177

R

racing thoughts 124–125, 126, 131
reading, bedtime 187
red light 43, 45, 49
relaxation strategies 35, 80–81,
    93, 111, 131, 133
REM (rapid eye movement) sleep
    17, 28–29, 30, 47, 52, 54, 55,
    59, 70, 91, 94, 117, 118, 121, 123,
    128, 131
  REM rebound 118, 157
restless legs syndrome (RLS) 57,
    72, 94, 95
restricting sleep 133, 139

S

seasonal affective disorder (SAD)
    172, 173
serotonin 23, 26, 88, 106, 131,
    152, 156, 173, 177
sex life 214–215
  orgasm 88–89
shift work 139, 146–147, 149, 204,
    216
short sleepers 17, 202
sleep
  functions of 14, 15
  sleep science discoveries
    16–17
sleep debt 53, 142, 143, 144
  catching up on sleep 142–143,
    196
sleep deprivation 48, 53, 58, 204,
    205, 210, 211, 214, 216
  cognitive performance and
    200–201
  impacts on health 196–197,
    202, 203, 207
  symptoms 196
"sleep drunkenness" 150
sleep efficiency 33, 36, 183
"sleep gate" 24, 25
sleep hygiene 34–35, 133
sleep inertia 29, 139, 150
sleep latency 33
sleep paralysis 70–71
sleep pressure (Process S) 16, 24,
    25, 43, 45, 82, 108, 128, 164,
    204, 214
sleep requirement 18–19, 33, 202
  by age group 18, 19, 62
sleep-tracking devices 33, 167,
    186

CREDITS

91 Leproult, R., Van Cauter, E., Effect of 1 Week of Sleep Restriction on Testosterone Levels in Young Healthy Men. JAMA 2011 Jun 1; 305(21): 2173–2174; DOI: 10.1001/jama.2011.710

92 Finan, P. H., Goodin, B. R., & Smith, M. T. (2013). The association of sleep and pain: an update and a path forward. The journal of pain : official journal of the American Pain Society, Dec 2013; 14(12), 1539–1552. DOI: 10.1016/j.jpain.2013.08.007

101 Erland LA, Saxena PK. Melatonin Natural Health Products and Supplements: Presence of Serotonin and Significant Variability of Melatonin Content. J Clin Sleep Med. 2017 Feb 15;13(2):275-281. DOI: 10.5664/jcsm.6462

116–117 Raphael Vallat, Postdoctoral fellow Walker Lab, UC Berkeley; The Science of Dream Recall, July 2019; raphaelvallat.com/dreamrecall.html

135 Maren J. Cordi, Angelika A. Schlarb, Björn Rasch. Deepening Sleep by Hypnotic Suggestion. SLEEP, 2014; DOI: 10.5665/sleep.3778W

SOURCE MATERIAL
To access a comprehensive list of source materials, studies, and research supporting the text in this book, please visit:

www.dk.com/science-of-sleep-biblio

About the author

Heather Darwall-Smith left a career in design to become a qualified psychotherapist, and has a diploma in Counselling and Psychotherapy and training in CBTI. She is currently working on a PGDip in Sleep Science at the University of Oxford. Heather believes that the path to well-being lies in a good night's sleep, and alongside her work as a sleep therapist at The London Sleep Centre, Heather runs a private practice online and in Oxford.

AUTHOR'S ACKNOWLEDGMENTS

I was discussing an idea with a wonderful colleague and friend, Dr. Petra Hawker, when she suggested it would make a fantastic subject for a book. Incredibly, DK agreed, and I cannot thank Dawn Henderson and Rona Skene enough for this opportunity; Rona in particular is an absolute superstar. My editor Aimée Longos is a miracle worker, and designer Alison Gardner and illustrator Owen Davey have both done a brilliant job of bringing my words to life visually.

To the London Sleep Centre team—Dr. Irshaad Ebrahim, Dr. Karina Patel, Stevie Williams, Rosie Musgrave, and Hayley Pedrick—thank you. To my clinical supervisor, Janet Croft, for your unfailing support, I can never thank you enough. I have also appreciated the help generously given by so many in the field of sleep science: Jesse Cook, Dr. Jade Wu, Dr. Christian Benedict, Sophia Pereira, and Professor Allison G. Harvey—thank you for responding to my various questions. Thank you also to Dr. Robin Darwall-Smith, Dr. Peter Gilliver, Anna Menzies, Lorna Ely, David Yaffey, Dr. Rachel Wood, Lisa Green, and Glynis Freeman, who all played an important role in my writing process and encouraged me to keep going.

Lastly, to Tim and Harry: none of what I do is possible without your relentless love and support; it's been another adventure on our great journey through life together.

PUBLISHER'S ACKNOWLEDGMENTS

DK would like to thank John Friend for proofreading, Marie Lorimer for compiling the index, and Deepak Negi for data permission clearing.

A NOTE ON GENDER IDENTITIES

DK recognizes all gender identities and acknowledges that the sex someone was assigned at birth based on their sexual organs may not align with their own gender identity. People may self-identify as any gender or no gender (including, but not limited to, that of a cis or trans woman, of a cis or trans man, or of a nonbinary person).

As gender language and its use in our society evolves, the scientific and medical communities continue to reassess their own phrasing. Most of the studies referred to in this book use "women" to describe people whose sex was assigned as female at birth and "men" to describe people whose sex was assigned as male at birth.